T3-BSJ-170

DYNAMICS of Family Development

PERSPECTIVES ON MARRIAGE AND THE FAMILY
Bert N. Adams and David M. Klein, Editors

WIFE BATTERING: A SYSTEMS THEORY APPROACH
Jean Giles-Sim

COMMUTER MARRIAGE: A STUDY OF WORK AND FAMILY
Naomi Gerstel and Harriet Gross

HELPING THE ELDERLY: THE COMPLEMENTARY ROLES OF INFORMAL NETWORKS AND FORMAL SYSTEMS
Eugene Litwak

REMARRIAGE AND STEPPARENTING: CURRENT RESEARCH AND THEORY
Kay Palsey and Marilyn Ihinger-Tallman (Eds.)

FEMINISM, CHILDREN, AND THE NEW FAMILIES
Sanford M. Dornbusch and Myra F. Strober (Eds.)

DYNAMICS OF FAMILY DEVELOPMENT: A THEORETICAL PERSPECTIVE
James M. White

DYNAMICS of Family Development

A Theoretical Perspective

James M. White, PhD
University of British Columbia

Foreword by **Roy H. Rodgers**

THE GUILFORD PRESS
New York London

A Division of Guilford Publications, Inc.
72 Spring Street, New York, NY 10012

Printed in the United States of America

This book is printed on acid-free paper.

Last digit is print number: 9 8 7 6 5 4 3 2 1

Library of Congress Cataloging-in-Publication Data

White, James M., 1946–
Dynamics of family development : a theoretical perspective/ James M. White.
p. cm.—(Perspectives on marriage and the family)
Includes bibliographical references and index.
ISBN 0-89862-080-5
1. Family. 2. Family—Mathematical models. I. Title. II. Series.
HQ503.W69 1991
306.85—dc20 91-9053
CIP

Cover design and pictogram by Otto Sanchez.

To Robin, Amy, and Kelly

Foreword

The first modern formulation of the family development theoretical approach was produced in 1948 by Duvall and Hill. Nearly 40 years later Mattessich and Hill (1987) published a major statement of the contemporary state of the approach. This work included a detailed "genealogy of evolving family development frameworks" with five major lines of intellectual ancestors: those who developed systems of life cycle categories, social system theorists, human development theorists, life span and life course theorists, and life events and life crisis theorists. Mattessich and Hill state that this "genealogical tree . . . has identified the diverse ancestral origins of the concepts and assumptions that make up contemporary family development as a theoretical orientation" (1987, p. 440). I am compelled to observe that only someone with the encyclopedic intellect of Reuben Hill would be capable of identifying in such detail the intellectual heritage depicted in those pages. Had he lived, I have no doubt that he would have continued his attempts to bring them together in a more unified theoretical structure.

Nevertheless, a candid look at the work of most of those who have identified themselves as "family development theorists" finds that they have worked in a much more restricted intellectual range—the one that traces its roots to life cycle category, social system, and human development theorists. Indeed, one of the continuing frustrations for many has been the inability to incorporate with any degree of comfort the ideas derived from the life span and life course theoretical area, Hill and Mattessich's 1979 efforts notwithstanding. A more minor focus has been the limited incorporation of the life events and life crisis theorists—a "marriage" that would also seem not yet to have been consummated! Indeed, the major work produced in the two decades that followed the first publication of Duvall's *Family Development* (1957) drew minimally from the theorists of life span, life course, life events, and life crisis. The publications dating from Hill and Rodgers (1964) to Aldous (1978) concentrated heavily on the elaboration and fine-tuning of a conceptualization whose roots were firmly in those three initial intellectual streams.

The 1960s and '70s were periods of high theoretical activity, along with empirical work that examined both the family dynamics over the family career and those aspects of family behavior that might be accounted for by the family life cycle stage.

Family development was not without its critics—both of the theoretical and empirical work. Mattessich and Hill (1987, pp. 460–465) effectively summarize these criticisms and provide their own limited responses. Of major import, however, was the explicit assertion of Holman and Burr (1980) that the family development approach should be labelled a "minor" approach because it had fallen into disuse in the previous decade. In my view, this evaluation was more accurate as a prediction of the decade to come than as a description of the decade just concluded. While Mattessich and Hill's work (1987) was important for its historical perspective and consolidation of the theoretical efforts of the previous 40 years (and more!), it did not serve to move the theory or empirical work much beyond where it had been at the end of the 1970s. They seemed unable to generate either productive theoretical propositions or significant empirical findings. While the formulation remained a convenient descriptor of family experience, almost metaphorical in character, it did not produce a model of family development with explanatory promise. Family development theory had apparently fallen into a moribund state in the 1980s.

I say "apparently" because, in fact, there *was* work being carried out which I believe holds the promise of a revitalization of family development theory. You hold in your hands the result of that work—though, as you will see, it is not nearly finished. It introduces a new "strain" in the genealogical chart—that of event history analysis as conceptualized by Coleman (1981), Featherman (1980; 1985), and Tuma and Hannan (1984). This work is combined with a "recessive" idea first introduced to family development by Magrabi and Marshall (1965) and which I picked up, but did not develop, in 1973: the stochastic nature of the family development process. When White creates his own fertile blend of these ideas and many of those already contained in the Mattessich and Hill genealogy, a considerably revised and, I believe, stronger theory of family development emerges.

White accomplishes a great deal in these pages. They can be summarized as follows:

1. He reviews and reformulates the theoretical literature on family development in a succinct and significant way.

2. He clarifies a number of previously vague and ambiguous principal concepts of family development theory. Perhaps most vital is his specification of the meaning and significance of the stage concept in family development theory. A major consequence of this is a radical

redefinition of this heretofore problematic idea. His extensive analysis in Chapter 11 of the centrality of the stage concept takes us beyond event history analysis and provides a clear direction for further theoretical and empirical work on the family career.

3. He clearly identifies the limits of applicability of family development theory. Mattessich and Hill (1987, p. 441) make reference to the "intellectual imperialism and eclecticism" in the history of the family development approach. White draws back from the "imperialism" in favor of a much more modest set of theoretical objectives, which strengthens the power of the theory in my view.

4. He provides new lucidity to the nature of family development as he draws on other behavioral science literature not previously employed.

5. He presents a theory that truly focuses on the *family* level of analysis—in its group, institutional, and aggregate forms. Of special note here is his introduction of a major new emphasis for our theoretical understanding that concentrates on the nature of the family career itself, rather than on families experiencing a stage or stages of their particular family career.

6. He produces a formal model of family development that is understandable to the mathematically unsophisticated (among whom I number myself), as well as the sophisticated. For the members of *my* group, I want to emphasize that understanding the abstract formulas related to the model is *not* required to comprehend it. On the other hand, I am sure that those who work with formal mathematical models will be stimulated to pursue the implications for family development that White has identified.

7. He specifies the methodological requirements for empirical testing of the theory and model.

8. Finally, and most significantly, he illustrates the model by applying it to data. He has thus met a rather rigorous set of criteria for theorizing, which he establishes early in the book. These criteria are demanded by the "theory–model–data triangle" discussed by Leik and Meeker (1975).

I have said that White presents in this work a major reformulation of family development theory. In the process, he has abandoned some aspects of the theory that others hold central. Other elements have been significantly reshaped. He has done so, however, on explicit theoretical grounds with the goal of increasing the explanatory power of the theory. There are those who will disagree with his reformulation. I am hopeful that White's work will precipitate vigorous theoretical and methodological discussion of the nature of family development. For I am certain that such debate will serve to further our understanding of the family career.

We are in the first year of the last decade of the 20th century. (I belong to that school of thought which holds that decades begin with the digit "1" and not "0"!) In my opinion White's work represents a genuine breakthrough for family development theory. To use the language of this reformulated theory of family development, this book is a *transitional event* that takes us into a new *stage* of theoretical development in the study of the family career.

Roy H. Rodgers
University of British Columbia

REFERENCES

Aldous, J. (1978). *Family careers: Developmental change in families*. New York: Wiley.

Coleman, J. S. (1981). *Longitudinal data analysis*. New York: Basic.

Duvall, E. M. (1957). *Family development*. Philadelphia: Lippincott.

Duvall, E. M., & Hill, R. (1948). *Report of the Committee on the Dynamics of Family Interaction*. Washington, DC: National Conference on Family Life.

Featherman, D. L. (1980). Retrospective longitudinal research: Methodological considerations. *Journal of Economics and Business, 32,* 152–169.

Featherman, D. L. (1985). Individual development and aging as a population process. In J. Nesselroade & A. Von Eye (Eds.), *Individual development and social change: Exploratory analysis* (pp. 213–241). New York: Academic Press.

Hill, R., & Mattessich, P. (1979). Family development theory and life span development. In P. Baltes & O. Brim (Eds.), *Life span development and behavior, Vol. 2,* (pp. 161–204). New York: Academic Press.

Hill, R., & Rodgers, R. H. (1964). The developmental approach. In H. Christensen (Ed.), *Handbook of marriage and the family* (pp. 171–211). Chicago: Rand McNally.

Holman, T. B., & Burr, W. R. (1980, November). Beyond the beyond: The growth of family theories in the 1970s. *Journal of Marriage and the Family, 42,* 729–742.

Leik, R. K., & Meeker, B. F. (1975). *Mathematical sociology*. Englewood Cliffs, NJ: Prentice-Hall.

Magrabi, F. M., & Marshall, W. H. (1965). Family developmental tasks: A research model. *Journal of Marriage and the Family, 27,* 454–461.

Mattessich, P., & Hill, R. (1987). Life cycle and family development. In M. B. Sussman & S. K. Steinmetz (Eds.), *Handbook of marriage and the family* (pp. 437–469). New York: Plenum Press.

Rodgers, R. H. (1973). *Family interaction and transaction: The developmental approach*. Englewood Cliffs, NJ: Prentice-Hall.

Tuma, N. B., & Hannan, M. T. (1984). *Social dynamics*. New York: Academic Press.

Preface

This book is a refinement and extension of the theory of family development. Substantively, the book is about the myriad of ways in which families traverse their life course. First and foremost, however, it is intended as a statement of the theory of family development that will be useful for graduate students and scholars studying the family.

The statement of the theory in this work is neither finished nor complete. Rather, in these pages, the reader is invited to participate in an ongoing process of theory construction and formulation. Indeed, I regard the version proposed here as not the only possible formulation of the theory of family development. This process of theory construction and formulation is less guided by social-psychological principles than most previous statements of family development theory have been. Rather, I have adopted somewhat different emphases.

Throughout this work, I have kept an eye on the theory's applicability to cultures and historical periods other than our own. Furthermore, I have accepted the notion that the theory of family development should not be isolated from the study of kinship. I believe these considerations have assisted me in developing a theoretical formulation that is not restricted to North American families in the 1990's or any other specific decade.

In formulating the version of the theory found in these pages, I have attempted to be precise—not simply through a careful and stipulative use of theoretical terms, but also through the formalization of theory. What I meanb by "formalization" of a theory is the transformation of the concepts and relations of the theory into mathematical terms. This allows a very precise and succinct statement of the major theoretical propositions. I hasten to add that although there are some formulas in this book, it is not a work designed for mathematically sophisticated readers. I have referred such readers to other works containing more detailed discussions of the models cited here. I have also attempted to make clear to nonmathematical readers the meaning and importance of the models to the theory and data analysis. Indeed, the book is largely addressed to this nonmathematical audience.

The impetus for this book came from my perception that three major areas of progress in the social sciences over the last two decades have a direct bearing on the theory of family development. First, social scientists have become increasingly aware that the family can be discussed on several different levels. These different levels of analysis require separate theoretical and conceptual treatment, since theoretical statements and concepts appropriate at one level may not be appropriate at another level. The second area of progress is recognition of the role of mathematical models in theory construction. Although previous authors had discussed "models" of family development, I did not fully perceive how such models fit together with theory and data until I encountered a discussion by Leik and Meeker (1975). The formalization of theoretical propositions appeared to me to offer the greatest promise for progress in constructing social-scientific theory.

The third area of progress in the social sciences that has suggested reformulating the theory of family development is the refinement and application of dynamic modeling, especially the "semi-Markov model." Although this model was introduced to many of us by Coleman (1964), it was not until the more recent works by Coleman (1981) and Tuma and Hannan (1984) that its implications for the analysis of retrospective family data became understood. However, the idea that the theory could be formalized by this model depended on the insight of Featherman (1985) that development is a duration- and state-dependent process. His insight ties the conceptual area to the semi-Markov model and suggests the formalization of the theory.

Although several of the chapters in this book analyze data relevant to the theory, these data should be seen as illustrations of elements of the theory rather than as empirical confirmation of the theory. Indeed, the chapters containing data analyses should not be viewed by readers as only "empirical" chapters. These chapters are very important ones for the extension of the theory into new areas. They should therefore be read as theoretical chapters, even though they contain more substantive material than the earlier "theoretical" chapters.

As with all projects such as this, there is a long history preceding the final product. In this regard, I would like to acknowledge several people as being particularly important to the completion of the project. Lyle Larson originally encouraged me to present a paper in this area in 1976. The late Reuben Hill was very supportive of my initial work in this area, and I doubt I would have ended up spending more than a decade on these ideas if it had not been for his encouragement. Robert Leik not only provided some of the material necessary for understanding the role of models in theory construction, but also read and commented on the first draft of the first two chapters. His comments and support are most appreciated. It is evident from Chapter 2 of this book that I owe both Bob Leik and Barbara Meeker an intellectual debt. During the writing of the first draft, Richard Jung, director of the Center for Systems Research at the University of Alberta, took time out of a busy schedule to read and respond to the first four chapters. Our long discussions at the center were especially critical to the development of the remainder of the book. Long-time friend and colleague Anthony Sims provided guidance in clarifying many of the concepts.

Also, I gratefully acknowledge the support I received from the Social Sciences and Humanities Research Council of Canada (Grant Nos. 410-82-0733 and 410-87-0141). Niall Trainor served as a diligent and creative research assistant. The University of British Columbia kindly granted me a sabbatical leave for 1987–1988, during which time I wrote the first draft of the book. I further acknowledge the assistance of Bert Adams and David Klein, editors of the Guilford Perspectives on Marriage and the Family Series.

A special acknowledgment must go to Roy H. Rodgers. His 1973 version of the theory has been immensely helpful to this formulation. In many regards, I see the work in this volume as a direct extension of Roy's 1973 book. Over the years, Roy has offered nothing but the best of scholarly and collegial assistance to me as I struggled with many theoretical wrong turns and dead ends. His careful reading of the first draft, and the many questions, comments, and corrections he made, have influenced much that the reader finds here.

Lastly, I would like to thank members of my family for their tolerance, understanding, and encouragement throughout this project. Special thanks to Robin, who edited portions of the manuscript while breastfeeding our daughter. And thanks to Amy and Kelly, who always renewed my enthusiasm for this project.

JAMES M. WHITE
Vancouver, B.C.

Contents

PART I

INTRODUCTION

CHAPTER 1

General Overview

We all know that individuals age, mature, and change throughout their lives. It may be less obvious, however, that social groups experience similar processes during their existence. A social group naturally changes with time, as does everything; this in itself is an unremarkable insight. What is more interesting is that social groups experience processes similar to the processes of aging and maturation for individuals. Indeed, the experience of the group is an important component in the individual's experience and growth.

This book examines the process of change in one particular social group, the family. The family occupies a unique niche among social groups. It is the most intimate of all social groups. It is a group that shares a common living arrangement. It is also a group that endures over a long period of time. And it is a group that is regulated by its own particular institutional norms—that is, the norms of the institution of the family. The unique character of the family suggests that the processes the family experiences are probably unique as well.

The processes of family change explored in this book are viewed from a particular perspective. That perspective is the theory of family development. Of all the extant theories about the family, the theory of family development is the one that has consistently emphasized the processes of change within families. This theoretical framework has a lengthy history, starting with the seminal development by Duvall and Hill (1948). Although the present discussion is not intended to be a thorough history of the theory of family development, a brief mention of the major contributions leading up to this work may be helpful.

Among the many contributions made to this theory by Reuben Hill, the book chapter coauthored with R. H. Rodgers (1964) entitled "The Developmental Approach" stands as one of the pivotal contributions to the theory. Indeed, some scholars view the Hill and Rodgers (1964) chapter as the "classic" formulation of the theory. Its ideas were further developed and refined in the book by Rodgers (1973). Two specific contributions that Rodgers (1973) made were to recognize the importance of levels of analysis in discussions of family change and to discuss the "family career" rather than the "family life cycle." Later, Aldous (1978), in her book *Family Careers,* reformulated much of the previous work on the family life cycle into the more sequential notion of the family career.

The most recent statement of the theory is the book chapter "Life Cycle and Family Development" by Mattessich and Hill (1987). This work contains an excellent overview of the historical antecedents and maturation of the theory of family development, including a complete list and discussion of the scholars influencing the theory. Since it is not the purpose of this book to review this history in depth, independently of any substantive question, interested readers are referred to the Mattessich and Hill (1987) discussion. In the present work, various contributions appear in the context of a particular discussion where they are important to a specific formulation, such as, for example, the specification of the process of development (Rodgers, 1973; Borne, Jache, & Sederberg, with Klein, 1978; Coleman, 1981; Featherman, 1985; Tuma & Hannan, 1984).

The theory of family development, as presented here, is both an extension of previous statements of the theory and a reformulation of some of the most basic concepts (e.g., the process of development). To some readers, the theory presented in this book may appear to be so distinctly different as not even to be considered the same theory as that developd by Duvall and Hill (1948). Indeed, the theory presented here has undergone significant revision in light of developments in contemporary social science. The broad outline of these revisions is discernible from the forces that have shaped them. First, the notion of "development" has become better defined (Featherman, 1985) and separated from other forms of change in families. Second, there is a much greater emphasis on identifying and specifying the process of development through using the process models discussed by Coleman (1981) and Tuma and Hannan (1984). Third, there is a greater emphasis on specifying the level of analysis to which theoretical statements pertain. Fourth, there is an increased emphasis on sequencing norms, rather than on the norms for behavior within a particular family stage (Hogan & Astone, 1978) Both Rodgers (1973) and Aldous (1978) have provided ample discussions of stage-specific norms. Scholarly progress in these areas has resulted in both additions and revisions to the theory of family development. Although differences with previous statements of the theory are sometimes discussed, the major emphasis in this book is on presenting a relatively coherent version of the theory to readers at this point in its development.

Thus far, several basic concepts have been introduced, such as "process," "development," "family," "group," and "social institutions," with little in the way of definition or clarification. The remainder of this chapter attempts to do two things. First, it introduces several of the ideas that recur throughout this work and provides an overview of the issues to be discussed. Second, the organization and contents of each subsequent chapter are briefly discussed, so that readers have a general notion of the path traveled in this book.

ORIENTING CONCEPTS

Simply stating that the theory of family development is a theory about a particular form of social group, the family, leaves some vagueness about the focus of the theory and the larger context. For example, a theory about a social group might deal with the signs and symbols used within and between social groups; or it might examine the growth and development of the individual in the context of the social group; or it might explore the development and change of the social group over time. The last of these three possibilities is the particular theoretical niche in which the theory of family development operates. Undoubtedly, a complete explanation would encompass all three of these elements:

1. The *cultural system* of signs and symbols and the processes of change in these signs and symbols.
2. The *individual system* of biological and psychological growth and development.
3. The *social system* of interaction and behavior in groups and social institutions, and the processes of change within and between these groups and institutions.

This does not mean that what we say about the social system, and more particularly about the family group and the institution of the family, does not have ramifications for these other systems. Indeed, a complete social theory would encompass all three plus the interfaces between them (e.g., societal–individual, societal–cultural, and individual–cultural). However, before such a complete theory can be developed, there is a need to fill in each system with a more restricted theory. In the present case, the discussion is restricted to the social system, and in particular to the institution of the family and the family group.

The Family: Structure and Norms

Earlier, I have characterized the family as a particular form of social group. That characterization does not represent a definition of the family. Defining "the family" is fraught with difficulties, since almost everyone has his or her own ideas in this regard. The concerns guiding this definition of the family should be made explicit. First, "family" as a social group should be defined so that the definition is consistent with other theoretical work about family and kinship. Not all theoretical work is equal in this regard. There is a body of theoretical work about kinship and fertility that is both rigorous and predictive; this work originated with Lévi-Strauss (1949) and has been further developed by H. C. White (1963). The major assumption behind this body of work is that family and kinship represent an area of social life regulated by social norms, which are sometimes proscriptive and prescriptive. The main purpose of these norms is to regulate affinal relations (mating and marriage) so that consanguineal relations (blood relations) will link groups in a system of alliances. The importance of this insight is that whereas affinal relations define marriage and mating, consanguineal relations define the family, and both define kinship. Thus, the principal characteristic of the family group is the consanguineal bond.

Four separate forces further establish that the consanguineal bond is the central defining feature of the family. First, the notion that one cannot call something a family without the presence of a parent–child relation abounds in the literature on the family (e.g., Reiss & Lee, 1988). Second, in the last two decades, there has been a marked departure from the two-parent nuclear family as a family form. The awareness of the diversity of family forms has forced family scholars into abandoning a single modal view and definition of the family. If, for example, the relationship between a single parent and a child is not considered to constitute a family, then the meaning of the term becomes increasingly reserved for a historical phenomenon as family forms change. Third, the theory of family development has been restricted in its specification of stages of family because it has adopted a "normative" view of nuclear-family stages, rather than stages that could be applied to any family structure (e.g., single-parent families and remarried families). The fourth development suggesting that the parent–child relation is central to the definition of the family is that there is an increased awareness of generational as opposed to cohort influences transmitted within the family (e.g., Bengtson, 1975; Glenn & Kramer, 1987). The only way to distinguish generational from cohort influences in the family is to focus on the consanguineal bond.

Besides the parent–child bond, there are other elements defining the family. These other elements can be distinguished by examining the statement "The family is changing." This statement has two distinct meanings. One is that the family as a group is changing its *structure*. For instance, using the parent–child bond as a defining characteristic does not mean that the social group may not contain more than one such bond. In fact, the statement that the family is changing could mean that there is a change from two parent–child relations in the group to only one. Thus, one meaning for the statement "The family is changing" is that the membership of the social group is changing.

A second meaning for the statement "The family is changing" is that the social *norms* regulating the roles and behavior of family members toward each other are changing (Elder, 1978, 1987). For example, norms regulating the division of labor and parental discipline in the family have changed over the last 30 years. However, when the statement refers to changes in norms, the meaning of the term "family" shifts from the social group per se to the institution of the family. A "social institution" is composed of all the social norms regulating a relatively well-delineated area of social life. Hence, all the norms regulating family roles and relationships compose the "family" as an institution rather than as a group.

These two meanings of "family" are coextensive, in that the group is constituted by its organization (or structure) and its organization is constructed by the institutional norms. For example, in the area of prescriptive kinship, H. C. White (1963) demonstrates that the social rules generate the social organization. Thus, it is impossible to talk about the family without considering both its group nature and its institutional nature. Any definition of "family" must include both of these elements.

What is the family? The definition used in this work is as follows: *A family is an intergenerational social group organized and governed by social norms regarding descent and affinity, reproduction, and the nurturant socialization of the young*. This definition is discussed more fully in Chapter 3.

Levels of Analysis: Institutions, Groups, Relationships, Individuals

One of the implications of this definition of family concerns the levels of analysis that may be used to examine the family. The most obvious level of analysis is the group level. This level entails the membership and structure of the family, such as the number of parent–child relations. Another level of analysis is the institutional level, which entails the nonidiosyncratic norms that regulate family roles, role relationships, and the sequencing of family stages within a particular society. The institutional level of analysis is implied by the distribution of behaviors for an aggregate such as individual members of families (i.e., fathers, mothers, or children), or by an aggregate distribution of group behaviors for families. The conceptual apparatus for an institutional analysis is the concept of "norm" or a social rule. Thus, the two major levels of analysis for the family are the group and the institution. There are other levels, such as family relationships and individual members. Although a more detailed examination of this topic is found in Chapter 3, Table 1.1 may give some notion of how the different levels are related.

Table 1.1 suggests that for each level of analysis, certain concepts and measures are appropriate. The concepts and measures presented in Table 1.1 are not the only ones appropriate for these levels, nor are they necessarily exclusive to the level at which they appear in the table. For example, naturalistic observation may be used as a measurement technique at several of these levels of analysis. However, the importance of levels of analysis for the theory of family development is that statements regarding concepts and processes at one level of analysis may not be true for other levels. There are probably distinct differences between processes of development for individuals and family groups, because of the different structures of these units. The process of development at one level cannot be assumed to be characteristic of the process of development at another. A more detailed discussion of the levels of analysis, and of the appropriate concepts and measures for each level, awaits the reader in subsequent chapters.

TABLE 1.1. Levels of Analysis for the Family, and Examples of Some Related Concepts and Measures

Level	Concept	Measures
Individual	Marital satisfaction	Individual questionnaire responses
Relationship (e.g., sibling, parent–child)	Agreement	Difference scores
Family group	Cohesion	Observation of group togetherness
Institution	Norms for families	Aggregate behaviors for a social system

Family Transitions

Not all changes in families are transitions. A "family transition" is a change from one stage in a family's development to another stage. Both stages are part of a developmental process. Furthermore, the probability of a transition's occurring between any two stages is partially determined by the duration of time spent in the preceding stage, as well as by the nature of the preceding stage. More precisely, transitions are both stage-dependent and duration-dependent (Featherman, 1985).

Every family experiences stages of development. For example, family formation begins with the event of the first child's birth. The so-called "launching" stage is the period between the departure of the first child from the home and the departure of the last child. As a family moves through the stages of its life course, its structure and membership change. Concomitant with these structural changes in the family are changes in the rules governing the roles and role relationships in the family. So, for instance, the roles of mother and father are added to those of husband and wife with the birth of the first child. Therefore, stages are meaningful at both the group level (structure) and the institutional level (norms) of analysis. The relationship between group structure and norms is complex. The norms not only set what is expected for a particular group structure and its members; they also set the expectations for which structures are in the appropriate sequence and "on time" with other life events.

The concept of "stage" is, in fact, central to the theory of family development. A stage is a qualitatively distinct period in the life course of the family group. A stage is determined by both the group structure and the social norms of the institution of the family. The social norms regulate the role relationships and expectations within the family that are appropriate to both a given stage ("static" norms) and the appropriate sequencing and timing of stages ("processual" norms). For example, there are norms governing how family members behave at a given stage (static), such as the expectation that mothers will exhibit nurturant behavior toward newborns. There are also norms as to what stage may be expected next in the family's life course (processual), such as those learned in the rope-skipping rhyme, "First comes love, then comes marriage, then comes Suzie with a baby carriage."

In researching family stages, we must often rely on inferences from the individual as a unit of observation. However, because the unit of observation is the individual, we should not conclude that the level of analysis is also the individual. Rather, individuals' behaviors taken as an aggregate are a means of inferring the institutional social norms for the dyad and group. The most useful indicator of family stages is the experience of a family transition "event." A family event (or dyadic event) is experienced and reported by an individual; however, a family event is necessarily an indication of something that happened in the family, although experienced and reported by an individual. In fact, a family event is one boundary of a family stage. The transitions between stages are punctuated and indicated by events. The experience of a transition between family stages can thus be inferred from the individual's report of a family event. If we know which events are theoretically tied to which stages, then an event indicates either the beginning or the end of a stage. However, as we shall see, the theoretical specification of stages lags behind the methodology associated with event transitions.

The study of family transitions is the study of the movement from one family stage to another. Family events are used as indicators of stage transitions; for example, the birth of the first child marks the transition from a dyad to a family. Events are used to indicate the transition points between stages. Figure 1.1 depicts the relationship between transition events and stages.

The institution of the family contains the static and processual norms regulating family stages and family transitions. However, the institution of the family does not operate in a vacuum. Other social institutions, such as work and education, contain social norms regulating the behavior of individuals and groups relevant to their areas of social life. It would be naive to assume that the institutional norms of the family can or do operate independently of other social institutions' timing and sequencing norms. For example, imagine a society in which the institution of the family holds the norm that males should financially support their offspring. The educational institution in this society holds the rule that people must remain in school full-time until a certain age. The cross-institutional norm generated by the conjunction of these two institutional norms is that males should not have offspring until after a certain age. Thus, one particularly important area of institutional analysis is the coordination of timing and sequencing norms among the various

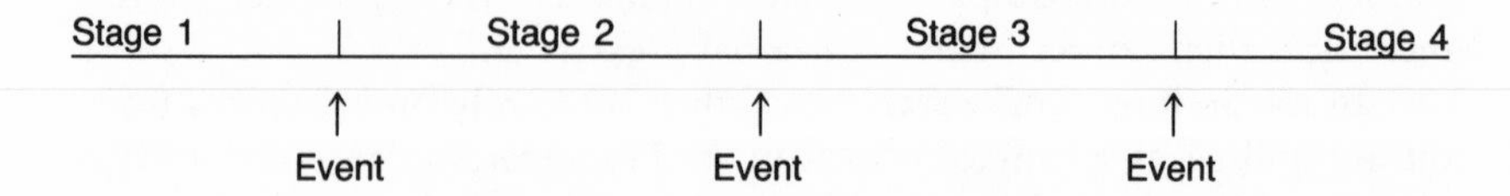

FIGURE 1.1 Relationship between stages and transition events. (Suggested by D. M. Klein, personal communication, 1988.)

social institutions. These cross-institutional norms are responsible for the synchronization of age-graded individual norms and stage-graded sequencing norms among social institutions.

So far, this discussion has introduced some of the concepts that are basic to the theory of family development: "norms," "family," "levels of analysis," "transitions," "stages," and "events." The discussion of these concepts also provides at least a hint of the direction of the theoretical formulation. With this basic picture in mind, readers can now place these concepts and the focus of this book within the framework of some of the basic questions facing the theory of family development.

BASIC PROBLEMS AND QUESTIONS

Several problems have hindered the advancement of the theory of family development. Fortunately, the basic problems have been succinctly summarized by Mattessich and Hill (1987, pp. 460–465), who identify four criticisms of the theory.

1. *A single modal life cycle?* The first criticism points to the fact that the stages used by theorists and researchers have largely ignored stages that would be relevant to remarried families or single-parent families. It is argued that the theory of family development focuses on one "normative" path of family development and ignores others. This problem can actually be broken down into several components. One possible reason for ignoring stages relevant to some families is that the definition of "family" used by theorists has been so restrictive as to exclude single-parent families. Another component of this criticism is that the theory of family development has failed to identify variations from the modal path as other than deviations from the set of stages that has become accepted as describing the "normal" or modal family career.

Mattessich and Hill (1987) state that this criticism has led to a re-evaluation of the descriptive adequacy of family stages and a move to enlarge the scope of family stages to become more relevant to other types of families, such as single-parent families. However, it is quite doubtful that simply enlarging the stages to describe more families at any point in time really addresses the crux of the issue (e.g., Hill, 1986). The real point is that the theory has not been sufficiently precise in its definition of family "stage." A precise analytic definition of "stage" would, in turn, allow any scholar to generate a possibility space for all possible family stages. What in fact has happened is that family scholars have attempted to construct analytic concepts from the "stages" they see in the empirical world, rather than to derive these analytic constructs theoretically. The result of this strategy is a set of stages restricted largely to one society and one point in history. The present work attempts to lay the foundation for an analytic treatment of family stages in Chapters 9, 10, and 11.

2. *Timing of critical life events.* Mattessich and Hill state that "A second, major criticism of the family development perspective has been that it ignores the timing of critical life events and the duration of stages, especially as these might be affected by historical context (see, for example, Elder, 1978)" (1987, pp. 461–462). This criticism also has several components. First, it is essential that the theory clarify and define the terms "stage" and "event" and the relationship between them. Second, it is an important aspect of this criticism that duration of time in a stage and the timing of stages have remained largely untouched by theorists in this area. Third, the relationship between time-related factors, such as age, cohort, and period effects, and the duration and timing of stages has remained unresolved by family-developmental theorists. This is linked in part to the overall criticism that these theorists have failed to identify and specify the exact *process* of change that they label "development." Also coupled with this is the criticism that the theory fails to discriminate the difference between other types of changes occurring in families and developmental changes. To sum up these criticisms, it would be fair to say that although developmental theory focuses on family changes over time, theorists have done little to refine the ideas of change and time within the framework of family development. Chapters 3 and 4 of this work attempt to identify and define these terms and the relationships between them.

3. *The interaction effect of other careers.* According to Mattessich and Hill (1987), the third major area of criticism is that the theory of family development has neglected the synchronization of the family career with other careers, such as work and education. They point out that stages in these other careers may precipitate transitions to new stages in the family life course. This criticism is only partially true. Aldous (1978) has dealt extensively with cross-career contingencies, and has even provided readers of her book with a suggestive table showing possible lagged contingencies among the family career, the educational career, and the occupational career. Furthermore, Hogan (1978) and many others working in the area of transition to adulthood have examined event sequences from various careers, such as first job, completion of school, and first marriage. Demographers of the family, such as Morgan and Rindfuss (1985), have also used event sequences. However, until the present work, much of this literature has not been integrated into the theory of

family development. Chapters 3 and 4 develop the theoretical underpinning for the analysis of cross-career contingencies in Chapters 9 and 10.

4. *Lack of correlation with other measures*. Finally, Mattessich and Hill (1987) state that the rather modest correlation with dependent variables leads many scholars to doubt that the theory of family development is much more than a descriptive device. Again, this criticism has several elements. First, many researchers have confused levels of analysis in their research. For example, some researchers examine family stages, a group-level phenomenon, expecting to find changes in marital satisfaction (an individual-level measure) without clarifying the theoretical linkage between group processes and individual outcomes (e.g., Klein & Aldous, 1979; Nock, 1979; Spanier, Sauer, & Larzelere, 1979). Second, since the theory of family development focuses on the process of development, but has as yet not clearly identified that process so that a test is indeed possible, any problems with "verification" of the theory must be seen as premature. In the present work, the model of development is specified in Chapter 5, and the assumptions of this model are empirically examined in Chapter 7.

Although this work does not claim to answer all aspects of the criticisms stated by Mattessich and Hill (1987), it does take these criticisms as highlighting major areas of the theory that need further specification and refinement. In this sense, this work builds on the work of previous scholars in the area. However, it seems that some of the solutions proposed to these problems necessitate dramatic changes in the theory. For example, as Mattessich and Hill point out, the process of development is not adequately expressed as simply one modal path. Rather, at each stage a family could make a transition to a less traveled stage and onto a less traveled family career path. This observation clarifies two things. First, variables within a stage may be relatively determinant of outcomes within that stage; as a consequence, causal and correlational analyses such as those commonly performed in the field may be justified. Second, although the variables within a stage may be deterministic, the paths that families traverse are not. These paths appear to be more accurately characterized as a stochastic process. Thus, the thinking becomes thinking about "dynamics" rather than "statics" and about "stochastic" processes rather than "deterministic" processes. This change in theoretical thinking is a departure from past formulations, although it has been hinted at by Magrabi and Marshall (1965), Rodgers (1973), Borne et al. (1979), Mattessich and Hill (1987), Elder (1985), and Hareven (1978). The movement of the theory into such areas as dynamic stochastic models and cross-career contingencies may seem to some scholars a break with the past tradition of this theory. I view this, however, as an extension and refinement of the theory of family development.

ORGANIZATION OF THE BOOK

The remainder of this book is organized into 11 chapters. Chapters 2 through 4 deal with relatively abstract concepts and assumptions. Chapters 5 and 6 introduce general problems in developmental methodology and the data sets to be used in the subsequent empirical explorations, respectively. Chapters 7 through 10 are concerned with expanding particular aspects of the theory and examining these ideas in an empirical light. Chapter 11 explores some of the broader implications and conclusions of previous discussions, in an attempt to expand the theory of family development to new areas. The final chapter, the epilogue, offers a perspective on the status of the theory of family development, as well as the strengths and limitations of the present work. Although most of the chapters stand as relatively independent statements, a perspective on the importance of each chapter to the overall project can only be gained by a complete reading of Chapters 2 through 5. These four chapters present the architecture of the theory. The other chapters serve to elaborate and expand the ideas introduced in Chapters 2 through 5.

Chapter 2 introduces the general view of science and theory that informs and guides the remaining chapters. It enunciates a position developed by Leik and Meeker (1975) that shows the complex relationships among theory, models, and data. This perspective is necessary in order to understand the importance of the formalization of theory into a model. Without this perspective, much of the discussion in Chapter 4 regarding the relation between the theoretical propositions and the model could be misunderstood.

A more detailed and elaborate discussion of the theory's basic concepts is provided in Chapter 3. Many of the concepts that have been introduced in the present chapter have been more emphasized here than in previous statements of the theory of family development. It is especially important that the concepts of "stage," "event," and "levels of analysis" be clearly understood, since these are used throughout this work.

The relationship between specific propositions in the theory of family development and the proposed model of the developmental process is explored in Chapter 4. The formalization of the theory in this chapter exposes many of the weaknesses in previous attempts to specify the theory. The most notable weakness is that the theory has yet to produce a set of developmental stages that would meet the logical criteria of being mutually exclusive and exhaustive.

Chapter 5 examines the many methodological problems in doing developmental research. The general theoretical problem of the lack of a set of specifiable stages is resolved by using events as indicators of transition points between stages. Thus, much of the empirical research to follow employs an event analysis approach. This chapter also serves as a general review of research designs for developmental processes.

The data collection procedures for the two data sets used in the empirical analyses are described in Chapter 6. The general parameters for each data set are described and compared, so that this material need not be repeated for subsequent chapters.

Chapter 7 examines the most critical assumptions of the model, the Markov and semi-Markov assumptions. More precisely, this chapter examines the duration- and state-dependent model for development, along with other competing models. The particular data used in this analysis are those for family formation (i.e., the probability of having a first child, given the previous childless state and duration in that state).

The affinal dyad or couple represents but one of the many possible sets of relationships in the family. Chapter 8 examines some of the processes in the affinal dyad as an example of research at the relationship level of analysis. Cohabitors and married individuals are compared on measures of marital quality, agreement, and individual perceived agreement. In addition, state and duration dependences for these measures are analyzed, in order to ascertain whether these dyadic measures are subject to developmental processes.

Institutional sequencing norms construct and influence the family career. These sequencing norms suggest which family stages are most appropriate along the family life course. Chapter 9 examines these norms to see whether there are gender and cohort differences in the sequencing of family events; it also examines some of the consequences for various sequences in later life.

Chapter 10 further develops the idea of deviance from the institutional norms for sequencing stages. An event analysis of both institutional and cross-institutional deviance examines differences in the consequences for each of these. Theoretically, this chapter develops the idea that processual deviance within one institution may be an adaptation to another set of institutional norms.

Chapter 11 presents a general overview and reassessment of the previous chapters. This chapter uses the empirical results of previous chapters both to illustrate and to re-examine the model and theory. The most important part of this chapter, however, is the attempt to develop a stage conception that satisfies logical criteria and is cross-culturally applicable. To demonstrate one consequence of this formulation, a measure of entropy is introduced to determine the degree of normative conformity in family stages and sequences between societies.

Chapter 12 is an epilogue. This chapter addresses the issue of the status of the theory of family development at this point in time. Areas of strength and weakness are discussed. This last chapter suggests areas for future research that are especially critical to the progress of the theory of family development.

One last general comment is in order before the discussion moves on to more detailed considerations. To date, most scholars working in the tradition of family development have referred to the theory as a "framework" or "perspective." Indeed, it seems as though these scholars have cautiously avoided calling this group of ideas a "theory" of family development. Perhaps such caution was justified in the past, but at the present time it seems that this theory is at least as well formulated as most of the competing theories about families. It is, therefore, the claim of this book that this represents *a theory* of family development. The next chapter attempts to define more clearly exactly what this claim of theoretical status entails, so that the reader may judge its accuracy.

CHAPTER 2

A Perspective on Science

At some point in the history of science, researchers might have been able to take for granted that their understanding of the scientific enterprise was shared by the colleagues who comprised their readership. However, Kuhn (1962) has brought this assumption of commonly shared definitions, methods, and understandings among members of the scientific community into question. This chapter, then, lays out the basic perspective on science that informs and motivates this work.

There are several reasons for making clear the assumptions behind this work, besides those implied by Kuhn (1962). First, the topic of family development is of interest to a broad range of scholars and practitioners. Not all of these readers are necessarily familiar with some of the more technical issues discussed in this work. Second, some of the terms used here, such as "theory," have received a myriad of definitions. It is therefore helpful to specify which of these meanings are implied in this work and which are not.

Another reason for making this perspective explicit is that this particular view of science guides this project in a "programmatic" way. The theory construction that this work pursues is directed by the understanding that the formalization of core theoretical propositions by means of a formal model represents a useful and appropriate way to proceed in developing and refining a theory. This view may be somewhat foreign even to those colleagues working within the substantive framework of family development.[1] Not all of these scholars are either familiar with or in agreement with the view that a substantive theory and an abstract model must be explicitly linked together in order to achieve the overall goals of scientific theory. However, this perspective on science is programmatic for this work. For these reasons, this chapter is devoted to a general explanation of this particular perspective on science.

THEORY

The term "theory" has a myriad of meanings in the social sciences. For some readers, a theory may mean mere speculation or conjecture, while for others it may imply a set of logically related statements with a truth value. For yet others, a theory is defined by its principal function of explanation (Homans, 1967). In this view, a theory should contain general statements linked together so that they explain some empirical event. Of course, then we can easily become immersed in the various interpretations of "explanation" and whether it is a psychological state or a formal characteristic of the set of statements. Instead of pursuing these various arguments in earnest, the strategy adopted here is to present the terms and meanings used in this work without becoming too embroiled in the complexities of philosophy of science. However, some of these arguments must invariably be addressed.

The first characteristic of the meaning of "theory" in this work is that it is not identical with "explanation." The term "theory" is used to mean a "scientific theory" rather than other types. In science, a theory is part of a larger architecture that provides explanation. That larger architecture is composed of the particular way human sensation is transformed into "data" and the particular way in which such "data" are considered to reflect or "model" the statements in the substantive theory. This complex architecture is composed of measurement typologies, mathematical models, substantive theoretical statements, and the rules of correspondence among the various elements in each. This complex architecture is discussed later in this chapter. For the moment, suffice it to say that, in this view, substantive theory alone does not provide explanation.

Rudner (1966) provides a definition of "scientific theory" that is a useful characterization. To quote Rudner (1966), a scientific theory is "a systematically related set of statements, including some lawlike generalizations, that is empirically testable" (p. 10). Three elements of this definition are essential for the meaning of "theory" proposed in this book. The first element is the meaning entailed by the phrase "systematically related set of statements." In this view, all the propositions of a theory should be linked, at least indirectly, to every other proposition. This logical linkage is what gives a theory its coherence and deductive power. Without this logical linkage, statements could exist that are ad hoc and arbitrary.

The second element in the definition that needs some interpretation is that a theory must contain some "lawlike generalizations." Lawlike statements are propositions with such empirical probability that they can be considered to occur invariably. Most lawlike statements are accompanied by the boundary conditions under which they hold, just as a parameter is a constant for a particular population. There are many such statements in the social sciences, such as "Families tend to follow the normative sequence of family events" (unless disturbed by other institutional norms or world events such as war or depression, or in other words *ceteris paribus,* "all else being equal").

The last element in the definition of "theory" essential to the meaning in this book is that theories must be "empirically testable." Following Popper (1959), many scholars might suggest that theories should be "disconfirmable." This may be too grand a claim for what is meant here by "theory." Even if one proposition does not hold empirically, there may be many explanations for this other than the falseness of the proposition. For example, the measurement typology may be inappropriate, or the sampling technique may have introduced errors into the data. What we can demand, however, is that a theory be empirically testable. That is, it should have some concepts that can be linked by rules of correspondence to a measurement typology or to direct sensation or observation. This point should become clearer in the discussions to follow.

MODELS

Like the term "theory," the term "model" has many different meanings in science. Indeed, many kinds of models are used in science. Among these are physical models, logical models, and mathematical models. For example, science often finds that physical analogue models are useful in such areas as understanding weather patterns or the structure of atoms. In the social sciences, the term "model" is primarily used to refer to mathematical or logical models. For example, the most simple measurement typology one can devise is one in which something is either present or not present. This is a binary measurement typology bounded by the assumptions of mutually exclusivity and exhaustive categories. Besides measurement typologies, mathematical models are commonly encountered in other areas of social science. In data analysis, we use mathematical models to find the best fit for the data. And in substantive theory, logical models are used to link propositions (systematic relations) or to present conceptual typologies. In this book, the term "model" is used to refer to this general type of use in the social sciences (i.e., mathematical models).

The most important point about mathematical models is that they are abstract and have no substantive content. It is important that mathematical models be content-free relative to both substantive theory and measurement, because the same mathematical model may be appropriate for very different theories and different data. In fact, one of the principal strengths of mathematical models is their generality, which is a result of their abstract character.

A mathematical model is composed of "variables," "parameters," and "operators." Variables are units that may vary; parameters are constants; and operators are rules of transformation. For example, the linear model $Y = a + bX$ contains Y and X as variables, a and b as parameters, and $=$ and $+$ as operators. The model transforms any given X so that it is equivalent to Y. This model could be part of a theory where income is said to be a direct function of education (concepts). This model could also be used to analyze data in a situation where a person's net income in dollars for a given year is related to the person's total years of institutionalized education (measures). In the theoretical example, the model formalizes a proposition in the theory, whereas in the data example, the model relates numbers of dollars to numbers of years of schooling. The elements of the model are content-free until we bring them into correspondence with an element of a theory (such as the concept "income") or an element of a measurement typology (such as "dollars per year").

DATA

The notion of "data" is central to empirical science. However, "data" do not have an independent existence out there in the "real" world; rather, like knowledge in general, they are products of human thought. There are no "facts" that exist independently of a system of assumptions that constitutes them as "data." Even the most simple data—those indicating presence or absence of an occurrence—entail assumptions regarding distinguishing one set from another, mutual exclusivity, and exhaustiveness. As an illustration, the observation as to presence or absence of children in a household presents many such problems of distinguishing between sets. Is the teenager who leaves home for work at a summer camp more "at home" than the child who died a week ago? Is the child who attends a residential private school and comes home on holidays living "at home"? What appears to be a simple measure in fact is a relatively complex series of decisions about set membership (presence or absence). These decisions regarding set membership should be guided by rules of inclusion that can be repeated by any independent researcher (replication). These rules should be part of the measurement typology. In addition, membership in one category should negate its being a member of the other category (mutual exclusivity), and the two categories should have to exhaust the possibilities for membership in the set (exhaustiveness).

"Data" are products of a measurement typology. A measurement typology at a minimum consists of rules of set inclusion, space exhaustiveness, and mutual exclusivity. This minimum constitution of data only provides categories and not continuous data. The familiar constructs of nominal, ordinal, interval, and ratio typologies often appear so automatic as to conceal the fact that each typology carries with it a set of assumptions that, when applied to our sensations, is as tenuous as any other hypothesis being tested. The notion of "facts" comes principally from the consistent use and consensual validity enjoyed by certain constructs (such as IQ), sometimes regardless of the adequacy of the assumptions underlying the typological constructs.

CORRESPONDENCE RULES

The relationship among theory, model, and data is a complex matter. For example, suppose we have deduced a simple theoretical proposition from a theory of marital relations stating that the duration of a marriage is inversely related to the quality of the marriage. The two concepts being related in this proposition are "duration of marriage" and "marital quality." If we decide to examine this proposition by conducting an empirical study, we must specify the exact relationship by using a model. So, for this example, the model could be a linear function such as $Y = a + (-b) X$. Once the model for the relationships is specified, we may begin to *operationalize* the concepts to be measured. However, the model itself further complicates this task, in that it constrains our selection of measures by limiting us to a level of measurement (measurement typology) where we can perform addition, subtraction, multiplication, and division. That is, the mathematical model constrains the operationalization of the concepts to variables measured at an interval level.

At each step in this example, there are rules of correspondence among the elements of the theory (concepts and relations), the elements of the model (variables and operators), and the elements of the measures (operationalizations, design, and measurement typology). We could continue with this example and follow the steps, returning to the theory once the data are collected; however, it is appropriate to turn to a more abstract and general treatment of this process.

It is apparent from this example that the correspondence rules among the elements of theory, model, and data are the key to arguments about validity, generalizability, and justification in science. The relationships among these elements are described by Leik and Meeker (1975). Leik and Meeker (1975) discuss correspondence rules as "mapping" one set of elements onto another. Since a mapping may not be symmetrical, the direction of the mapping makes a difference. For instance, a mapping of theoretical elements *onto* the elements of a mathematical model might mean that there would be more than one theoretical element mapped onto each element of the model. Ideally, one would prefer to have a single relation for every element of both theory and model, or an "isomorphic" correspondence. This ideal is not always possible.

Leik and Meeker (1975) illustrate the various correspondence rules or mappings among data, theory, and model in a diagram they call "the theory–model–data triangle" (see Figure 2.1). The following discussion explains each of the links among theory, model, and data identified in this figure.

In order to interpret Leik and Meeker's diagram, it is necessary to distinguish between "inductive" and "deductive" modes of inquiry. In a deductive mode of inquiry, one begins with general theoretical propositions, which then yield more specific expectations about the data. Induction follows the opposite path: Specific data are used to create more general statements. In Figure 2.1, each side of the theory–model–data triangle has both an inductive and a deductive component.

The relationship between theory and data (I4, D4) is one that is often acknowledged as paramount in regard to the scientific enterprise. The deductive mode (D4) represents the theoretical prediction of an observable outcome. The actual "deduction" may be a formal one or, as is more likely in the social sciences, simply a reasonable consequence of the theory.

The inductive mode of the relationship between theory and data (I4) involves the interpretation of the data. For example, the research finding of an increase in premarital cohabitation can be interpreted by the theory of family development as the evolution of a new stage in the courtship process of dating, engagement, and marriage. Although there is no logical necessity to this as opposed to any other theoretical interpretation, such interpretations often spark new hypotheses for further examination. An example of a new hypothesis derived from a theoretical interpretation is that premarital cohabitation is a transient stage often ending in marriage.

The relationship between theory and model (I1, D1; I2, D2) is more complex. In one direction, the theory is mapped onto the model (I1, D1). This is known as "formalization." The formalization of theory often requires a theorist to focus upon those elements of the theory that must be considered core or central, and those elements of the theory that are less so. What is achieved by the formalization of the substantive theory is a more abstract statement of the relations in the theory. This abstract picture of the theory can more easily be related (or generalized) to other theories sharing the same model or a similar model, since one is no longer sidetracked by the substance of the matter, but only faces the relations in the theory (I1). As we shall see in Chapter 5, formalization is very helpful in dealing with theories of process, such as the theory of family development.

The mapping of the model onto the substantive theory (I2, D2) provides the theory with the formal powers of the mathematical model

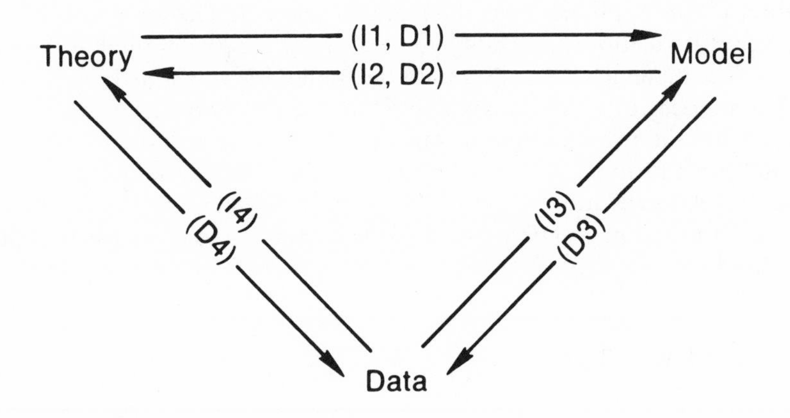

FIGURE 2.1. The theory–model–data triangle.
Inductive Modes:
I1—Mathematical generalization of theory.
I2—Substantive interpretation of mathematical patterns.
I3—Mathematical generalization of empirical patterns.
I4—Substantive interpretation of data.
Deductive Modes:
D1—Formalization of theory.
D2—Derivation of substantive hypothesis from mathematical patterns.
D3—Mathematical prediction or extrapolation.
D4—Substantive prediction.
The term "substantive" implies reference to a particular area of interest such as social mobility, small-group interaction, and the like.

From *Mathematical Sociology* by R. K. Leik and B. F. Meeker, 1975, Englewood Cliffs, NJ: Prentice-Hall. Copyright 1975 by Prentice-Hall, Inc. Reprinted by permission of the publisher.

in deducing substantive consequences (D2). Furthermore, the model may provide the theory with interesting mathematical patterns to interpret (I2). For instance, a discrete-state process model may provide the theory with such characteristics as an "absorbing state" in which the process stops. This formal characteristic challenges the substantive theory to provide a conceptual interpretation for this "absorbing state" in the model, such as "death" or "happiness."

The relationship between model and data (I3, D3) is a familiar one to most empirical researchers. The mapping of the model onto the data (D3) constrains the data, in that it must be organized to fit that particular model. For example, if the model is a simple linear model with two variables ($Y = a + bX$), then the data must be at the appropriate level of measurement, the relation must be linear, variances must be approximately equal, and so on. If one proceeds by mapping the model onto the data, the correct test is clearly a test of "best fit." To the degree that the model is an improbable fit, the model is rejected. The logic here is the reverse of the more usual null hypothesis tests at a particular alpha level.

The mapping of the data onto the model (I3) is distinctly different. Any number of models may be used in order to find the one that best describes the relations among variables. This is what Leik and Meeker call "curve fitting." In this enterprise (I3), the data may be mapped onto several different models until a "best fit" is found. This model, then, offers a mathematical description of the relations among variables in the data.

EXPLANATION

An explanation of a phenomenon is closely tied to theory. It is basic to the notion of "explanation" that it provides a reason why something happens. For example, Homans (1967) uses the example of explaining why water is sometimes warmer on one side of a lake than on the other, given the same amounts of exposure to the sun. His explanation includes the ideas that warm water rises to the surface, that winds move surface water toward one shore rather than the other, and that the water being moved is warm water. His example is useful in order to gain some general notion of explanation. However, it is a somewhat misleading example if it is thought to characterize scientific explanation. It is not misleading because it is wrong; rather, it is misleading because it is less than a complete picture of explanation in scientific inquiry.

Scientific explanation is not simply the interpretation of an event using some theoretical propositions (I4 in Figure 2.1). Rather, scientific explanation involves the elements of interpretation, prediction, precision, connectedness, and empirical validity. In fact, many of these elements are implied in Rudner's (1966) definition of scientific theory. Some of these elements need further clarification.

Every theory should be able to interpret events that are within its substantive venue. This means that it should be possible to select particular aspects of an event and to establish a correspondence between these aspects and concepts in the theory. Thus, when one is interpreting an event, one assumes that the empirical aspects are related in the same way as are the concepts in the theory. This is quite different from prediction (D4), in which certain conceptual hypotheses are derived from the theory and rules of correspondence are established between the concepts and the empirical measures. This task implies that equivalent relations among concepts must also be found among the empirical measures.

The idea that explanation is only explanation if the theory is considered to be valid leads to the relation between the model and the data (D3). The prediction from a theory can only be validated if we can analyze how well the data fit this particular theoretical model rather than the other possible ones. It is insufficient to assume that the inductive generalization of data to a model provides this kind of validation (I3). However, this may be a starting point for the development of theory. Validation is, of course, never complete and always a matter of probability.

The fact that a model is a necessary component for validation suggests that there needs to be a connection between the theoretical propositions and the model (I1, D1; I2, D2). On the one hand, this link provides a logical test for the theory. If the theory is inconsistent, too vague, or ambiguous, this will surface in the formalization of the theory (I1, D1). Leik and Meeker (1975) put it this way:

> A poorly delineated theory cannot provide adequate basis for developing a mathematical model; if modeling based on such a theory is attempted, it will soon become evident that the information contained in the theory is not sufficient to determine the properties of the variables or forms of relationships. (p. 227)

This statement may be seen by some scholars as indicating that only the most sophisticated social theories are ripe for formalization. However, another interpretation is that attempts at formalization will show the areas where the theory requires greater thought and specification. Hence, formalization is seen as a tool assisting in theory construction and refinement.

The last element that is expected in an explanation is a "connectedness" to other areas of thought. This point is often lost amidst the other criteria. It is essential that a theory be tied to other areas of thought. There are several ways for this to happen. One way is that some of the concepts in the theory appear in other substantive theories. Another way this happens is that the model is one used in other theories. In this sense, the same relations are invariant for several theories regardless of specific content. Where the model is one of a process, this may lead to insights about the nature of change in diverse areas. In this sense, the relations in the theory constitute a particular incidence of a more general and abstract system of relations in the model (I2, D2).

Explanation involves all of the elements and relationships in the theory–model–data triangle. To exclude any one of these elements is to truncate our capacity to understand our environment and ourselves.

THE DYNAMICS OF THEORY CONSTRUCTION

The foregoing discussion may leave the unintended impression that a scientific theory is a "product" to be scrutinized and evaluated by the criteria enumerated above. In the social sciences especially, much time has been spent in evaluating whether or not a set of ideas has attained the status of a scientific theory. However, the present discussion does not intend to encourage such evaluations.

As I see it, there are many possible social-scientific theories. The maturation and development of these into theories that are better approximations of explanations depends on the success in following the program implied by the theory–model–data triangle. For example, a theory with weak or imprecise systematic relations between its statements will be exposed as such when attempts at formalization are undertaken. Then, appropriate recasting will have to be undertaken. A theory with little, if any, empirical import will be revealed as such when one attempts to deduce predictions. Thus, the question for the social sciences seems not to be "Which of our theories have attained the status of a scientific theory?" but, rather, "What is the process by which we improve and nurture theories so that they come closer to scientific explanation?" Clearly, the first question is one about a "product," and the second question is concerned with the "process." The perspective taken in this book is that the theory–model–data triangle serves as a programmatic statement in regard to this process.

PROGRAM

The particular view of science outlined in this chapter suggests a program for approaching the development of theory. This book can best be understood as a work that follows this process. Many things are accomplished, but many more remain unresolved. This project is not aimed at producing the final statement of the theory of family development. It is aimed at nurturing and improving the overall state of the theory and the explanations it affords. This process can best be understood by keeping in mind the various dimensions of the theory–model–data triangle, since this perspective both informs and guides this work.

The program suggested by this particular perspective on science contains several aspects. First, some of the concepts in the theory of family development are clarified. The specification of the appropriate model for the process of family development assists in this task. Second, the most general and process-oriented theoretical propositions from the substantive theory are used to specify the particular model appropriate for that process. Third, the basic assumptions of the model for family development are discussed in relation to research design and methodology. Fourth, the most basic assumptions of the model are examined in light of empirical data. Fifth, some of the implications of the theory and model are pursued in the broader context of social institutions. And finally, the problems, limitations, and future directions of this theory are examined. In brief, this program is suggested and justified by the particular view of explanation and science developed in this chapter.

NOTE

1. See Burr (1970) for a more elaborate discussion of substantive issues.

PART II

THEORY

CHAPTER 3

Concepts in the Theory of Family Development

CHANGE AND DEVELOPMENT

All developmental theories—whether about individuals or families, organizations or populations—emphasize time as a crucial element. For example, cognitive development in individuals is often examined using Piaget's framework of irreversible, monotonic, and sequential stages of development (Flavell, 1963). Changes in families over time have been analyzed as stages in the family life cycle or family career (Aldous, 1978). The survival of business organizations has been examined as a function of time and complexity (Hannan & Freeman, 1984). Population dynamics are often analyzed as evolutionary changes brought about by selection and adaptation (Hawley, 1950). However, these examples and the many others that come to mind raise an important issue in regard to developmental theories. The issue in question is the distinction between all change in general and developmental changes in a unit. Clearly, if all one intends is that "development" and "change" are synonymous, then why bother with the possible obfuscation, let alone the terminological redundancy?

The only defensible answer to this query is that there is an important distinction between the meanings of the terms "development" and "change." Featherman (1985) addresses this question and offers an insightful distinction between the two:

> *Development* is one form of time-dependent change of the organism's state. This change can be quantitative, as in moving from one level of a continuous variable to another over some interval of observation; it may also be qualitative. The special feature which discriminates development from such generic quantitative and qualitative change in time is *duration dependence,* a characteristic of the rate of change. If the rate of leaving (or entering) a state is a function of the time spent in that state, then change is dependent upon duration. (p. 215)

The notion that development is one form or type of change that is identified by "duration dependence" implies that some forms of change are clearly not developmental. Furthermore, according to Featherman, developmental change implies that the probability of a transition to another stage is determined by the length of time spent in a stage.

A fairly obvious consequence of this definition of development is that states or stages tied to biological maturation are developmental and that such states are also correlated with chronological or birth age. Thus, as in many theories of individual development (e.g., those of Kohlberg and Piaget), stages are associated with the birth age of the individual because the duration of time in each state is relatively homogeneous across individuals. Featherman (1985) refers to transitions between these states as "age-graded transitions." The term can also refer to transitions between states in which the duration of time is set by the norms of social institutions. For instance, the duration of time spent in kindergarten is relatively stable, not directly because of biological maturation, but because educational institutions dictate the age at which children begin school. Nonetheless, the institutional norms are at least as closely correlated with chronological age (age-graded) as is biological maturation, if not even more so.

There is another type of transition between states that is duration-dependent and thus developmental. This is the type of transition between states in which the beginning of the process is not birth but some other event. Featherman calls this type of transition between states an "event transition." An example of a process involving event transitions is one in which the beginning is the onslaught of a disease. The probability of transitions to various outcome states (e.g., rapid recovery, prolonged illness, or death) is determined by the duration of time from the beginning of the disease. This notion also applies to many learning situations in which the time spent studying a subject is related to levels of mastery, as in mathematics. Still another example of such a process would be marriage, the duration of which determines the probabilities of divorce or having a child.

This last example, that of the duration of marriage, illustrates that many state-to-state transitions may exemplify both types of transitions. Duration of marriage and subsequent transitions to states such as divorce or becoming a family are determined by both chronological age (age-graded transitions) and time spent in marriage (event transitions). As an event transition, a wedding may be looked at as beginning the first stage in family formation; hence, it is logically the starting state from which duration of the marriage is reckoned. From this perspective, the time spent in marriage determines the probability of subsequent transitions, independently of chronological age. However, age-graded social norms may also determine the probability of subsequent transitions. For example, there are clearly age-graded social norms about the age range in which one should get married and should have a family. Thus, although these two types of transitions, age-graded and event, may be logically and theoretically separable, they are almost always empirically confounded. This problem is one to which we shall return in the discussion of methodological problems.

This view of development has several implications for the theory of family development. One implication is that development is a stochastic rather than a deterministic process. Some developmental theorists (e.g., Piaget, Freud) conceptualize development as a monotonic progression through successive states. One may be halted at a particular state, but usually the progression is seen as irreversible. The view of development outlined above suggests that the process is not characterized ipso facto by either reversibility or irreversibility. Rather, the identification of empirical processes that are developmental rests solely on the fact that these processes (whether they be cognitive or family or organizational) show that the *probability* of a transition to some other state is conditional upon the duration of time in the present state. The direction of the transition is not determined by this definition of development. Furthermore, this does not represent a deterministic statement, so it is a possibility that not all people will follow the transitions to the next most probable state.

LEVELS OF ANALYSIS

It is possible to discuss development as a process, abstracted from any particular unit or organization that is developing. However, it seems well advised to keep in mind that some *thing* always develops: an embryo, a human being, a family, or perhaps a social organization. What has become clear from the study of development in the biological sciences is that statements about one level of organization are not necessarily true of other levels. For example, statements about the development of a cell may include statements about DNA. However, the development of a cell in the organism must be treated as quite different from the development of the organism as a whole. An organism's development entails interactions with an environment that is quite different from the cell's environment, and the requisite structures for adaptation to environmental changes are likewise quite different. At some point, an organism's adaptation is assisted by learning, a characteristic not shared by cells except in the most trivial of ways. If we go up one more level to the population, processes are clearly unlike those at the cellular level. For any particular cell, it would be silly to talk of natural selection; however, for populations, natural selection is a key process to understanding how they change over time.

Sometimes it is possible to apply statements from more general levels of analysis such as the population to explain why individual members of the population do not survive, but the reverse of this does not seem to be true. In general, it appears that some statements at more general levels of analysis may be meaningful for subunits or lower levels of analysis, but that lower-level processes are seldom appropriate for higher levels of analysis. Whenever statements from one level are supposed to explain some phenomenon at another level, caution is warranted. The success of moving statements from one level to another rests on a careful examination of the theoretical connections between levels, as well as the unit of observation on which data are being collected. In regard to the unit of observation, every introductory text on methods contains illustrations and warnings in regard to the "ecological fallacy."

In their application of population ecology to organizations, Hannan and Freeman (1977) suggest that in regard to human organizations, more levels of analysis are required than the three levels of individual, population, and community normally used in population ecology:

> The situation faced by the organizations analyst is more complex. Instead of three levels of analysis, he faces at least five: (1) members, (2) subunits, (3) individual organizations, (4) populations of organizations, and (5) communities of (populations of) organizations. (p. 933)

Other theorists, such as Rodgers (1973), have suggested the three levels of individual, group, and institution as levels of analysis. However, the proposal by Hannan and Freeman has much to recommend it. In order to argue for the finer gradations they propose, it helps if the levels are proposed in terms of more usual sociological units.

The category of "members" in the Hannan and Freeman proposal clearly corresponds to "individuals." As a level of analysis, this is undoubtedly the most familiar, since this is the minimum unit for human social action or behavior. The second level of "subunits" is more difficult. Subunits must refer to those units that may be part of an "organization" but do not entail the characteristics of an organization. For example, the family contains many subunits, such as dyads (e.g., siblings, marital, and parental) and triads (e.g., siblings and parents–child). These subunits can be analyzed separately from the family, as is most often done with marriage; however, the analysis will necessarily miss the organizational context of this subunit, which is the family. The third level is the "individual organization." This would be, for example, the Jones family or the Smith family. The particular family, with its idiosyncratic rules of conduct and ways of seeing the world, is analyzed at this level. The fourth level is that of "populations of organizations." This level refers to "families" within particular parameters, such as geographic or ethnic. At this level, analysis concentrates on the variation within and between populations of families. An example of such a research question would be "Are black families in North America more matrifocal than are white families?"

The last level of analysis is "communities of organizations." A "community" implies not just a geographic communality but other common characteristics as well. These characteristics are usually shared understandings about behaviors appropriate to the organization. The term used by Rodgers (1973) for this level is "institutional." Rodgers views the institution of the family as analyzable as the aggregate of family behaviors. What is important is that at this aggregate level (e.g., families in North America), the behaviors indicate the norms or social rules that compose the social institution of the family. Following Bierstedt (1970), Rodgers (1973) offers the following definition: "[A]n institution is the set of rules which defines the way in which something ought to be accomplished" (p. 25).

Added to the idea that the institution is constructed of the social norms (rules) governing one particular area of social life, such as family life, religious life, or political life, is the notion that with these norms sometimes come sanctions that reward and punish families and individuals for not following the rules. As Rodgers (1973) puts it, even though there is some degree of ethnic and social class variation,

> Nevertheless, as one observes family life throughout the American culture, one finds a clear common thread of behavior running through it that is based on societal–institutional expectations about which all members of the society know and to which they conform to a considerable degree. (p. 24)

Thus, at the "communities of organizations" level lies the important sociological construct of "social institutions." This construct explains common behaviors between and within families as guided by the normative structure of the institution of the family.

The levels of analysis adopted for the present study of family development follow Hannan and Freeman (1977), with some minor modifications. The levels of analysis are (1) individuals; (2) family subunits; (3) family organizations; (4) aggregations of families partitioned by some characteristic, such as ethnicity or social class; and (5) the social institution of the family for a given culture, as indicated by the total aggregate.

THE FAMILY

One possible reason for the existence of so many definitions of the family is that any one definition may be concerned mainly with one or more levels. A definition of the family may be concerned with any of the levels of analysis defined above, particularly with the three following: (1) the family as an organization or group ("a family"); (2) the family as a population of organizations ("families"); or (3) the family as a social institution ("the family"). For example, some definitions emphasize the family as a collection of structured roles, stressing the organizational level (e.g., Parsons & Bales, 1955). Others emphasize the interacting personalities in the family, stressing the individual and subunit levels (e.g., Waller & Hill, 1951, pp. 25–36). And still others emphasize the institutional level of analysis, as, for example, Rodgers (1973) does in stating,

> The family is a semi-closed system of actors occupying interrelated positions defined by the society of which the family system is a part as unique to that system with respect to the role content of the positions and to the ideas of kinship relatedness. (p. 15)

Essentially, all of these definitions have in common at least some emphasis on the social organization of the family. This may be implicit, such as in the case where "interaction" implies the norms that construct the role relationships for interaction, or it may be more explicit, as in the Rodgers (1973) definition. It seems that the essential ingredients of a reasonable definition of the family should include the following three components: (1) the sector of social life that is organized; (2) the institutional nature of organizing norms; and (3) the nature of the group being organized. The following definition, first presented in Chapter 1, attempts to incorporate these ingredients: *A family is an intergenerational social group organized and governed by social norms regarding descent and affinity, reproduction, and the nurturant socialization of the young.*

In this definition, the sector of social life that is organized is that of affinal and consanguineal relationships, as well as the reproductive relationships of members of the society. Many definitions of the family do not consider the organization of kin relations, since modern North Americans tend to think almost exclusively of the conjugal family. However, if a definition of family is not supposed to be narrowly defined by the interests or trends of one historical period, then kin relations must be included on the basis of both ethnographic evidence and existing theory (e.g., Lévi-Strauss, 1949: H. C. White, 1963). The inclusion of reproduction and nurturant socialization seems noncontroversial since the work on the universality of the nuclear family (e.g., Murdock, 1949; Reiss, 1965).

The institutional nature of the organizing norms is more implicit in this definition than in some others. It is implicit that norms are social rules receiving authority from community agreement concerning the appropriate behavior in areas of social life. It is also implied that these social norms receive much of their force from the consensus from which they emerge, as well as from possible sanctions attached to compliance and noncompliance.

The last characteristic a definition of the family should have is a statement about the nature of the social group. The proposed definition characterizes the family as an intergenerational group. Thus, the minimum requirement for members of a family is that there be two members from different generations, usually a parent and a child. "Generation" is a term that may at times be confused with "age cohort." What is meant here is the more technical meaning as noted by Uslaner in the series editor's introduction to Glenn:

> The word *generation* is frequently misused. Technically it is a structural term derived from the parent–child relationship and should be reserved to that usage. Its other common use—to identify a group of individuals who are linked by age (the "Depression babies") or modes (the "Pepsi generation") or class (law students)—is correctly an identification of *cohorts.* (Glenn, 1977, p. 5)

The definition of the family proposed here views the nature of the group as intergenerational, meaning that there is either a biological parent–child relationship or a *fictive* parent–child relationship in the group. Without the presence of such a relationship, the group is not a family. Thus, calling a communal group or Charles Manson's group a "family" clearly violates the meaning of "family" as defined here.

Several implications follow from this definition of the family. One implication is that since a family contains a parent–child relationship, the institutional norms must fill in the social rules governing that relationship, such as the incest taboo, mating, and descent. Another important implication is that the core role relationship for the family is a parent–child relationship and not a marriage. This may seem an especially contentious claim if it is not clarified further.

There are two levels on which the present definition of the family might seem to imply that marriages are not families. At the *group* level, a family must contain a parent–child relationship. This means that marriages are a separate form of social group with a structure different from that of families. A marriage is defined by the affinal relationship between adults, whereas a family is defined by the consanguineal relationship between individuals of different generations. Hence, at the group level, the structural difference between a marriage and a family is quite clear.

Some confusion arises when moving to the *institutional* level and discussing the family. The institution of the family is composed of the social rules governing this area of social life. For centuries, marriage has served as a first step in the development of the family. People have married with the intention of having children. The central norms governing consanguineal relations, such as the incest taboo, also govern marriage and mate selection (Lévi-Strauss, 1949). So it is true that the norms within the institution of the family govern marriage, mate selection, descent, family, and kinship as one unified and intertwined system. Although the social group of the family is clearly different from the social group of marriage, it is impossible to differentiate many of the norms for marriage clearly from the norms for family. For example, norms governing marriage are usually contingent on the presence of children as well as the ages of the children. Sequencing and timing norms regarding marriage are tied to the biology of reproduction. And, for the great majority of marriages, even the solitary marital dyad is embedded in the system of extended family and kinship. Therefore, marriage and family can be viewed as distinct social structures at the group level; however, at the institutional level, there is only one system of social norms for the institution of marriage, family, and kinship.

THE THEORY OF FAMILY DEVELOPMENT

Most theories contains elements of both static analysis and dynamic analysis. Usually one of these two elements receives greater attention than the other. For instance, if a theory is concerned with explaining and describing family organization, a static or synchronic analysis may be justified. However, if a theory is concerned with changes over time in family organization, a dynamic or diachronic analysis is warranted. Naturally, some of the concepts appropriate for one approach may prove useful in the other approach. But some concepts are necessarily unique to each one, especially to dynamic analysis.

A theory of family development is clearly concerned with explaining patterned changes in families over time, and hence emphasizes dynamics. In many of the previous efforts at formulating a theory of family development, however, a static analysis has occupied center stage. For example, Rodgers (1973) relies on Bates's (1956) work on roles and role structures to introduce the core concepts of his version of a theory of family development. He then posits that these structures change over time, but fails to specify the *process* by which they change. Aldous (1978) adopts a similar approach. These efforts have largely addressed the role and position structures in families. However, it seems that a theory of family *development* should emphasize dynamic analysis in its perspective on how families change over time.

Having said this, I should note that previous attempts at a theory of family development are *not* bereft of any reference to changes in families over time. One key concept has emerged as central to the dynamic formulation of a theory of family development: the notion of "career." Rodgers (1973, p. 19) introduced this concept of "family career" as meaning all the various role clusters at each point in time tied together sequentially over the life of the group. Aldous, in her 1978 book *Family Careers,* uses a similar definition. However, she too develops her notion of the family career from a static analysis of roles and positions *à la* Bates (1956). The following passage illustrates how time is simply thrown into the static analysis to add the essential ingredient of development:

> The concepts of role sequence, role cluster, and positional career are interrelated to and interdefined with the concepts of role, norm, and position from which they stem. Thus, *when given a time dimension,* the idea of role cluster suggests the need of the concept of positional career just as the concepts of role, *when viewed from a temporal perspective,* gives rise to the concept of role sequence. (Aldous, 1978, p. 12; italics added)

These theorists have, however, launched the concept that is the core construct for a dynamic analysis of family development—the family career.

The starting point for the construction of a theory of family development necessarily returns to the previous discussion of levels of analysis. The fifth level of analysis set forth there is that of the institution of the family. The institution of the family is composed of the commonly agreed-upon social norms regarding family life (e.g., descent, affinity, reproduction, socialization). Although social scientists often assume a common understanding of social norms, it is worth being clear in this regard.

A social "norm" is a social rule. A "rule," following Black (1962), is a commonly agreed-upon relationship between an act, a position, and a modality. Every society is composed of social positions that are given like points in the social structure. These positions are analytic, in that they may be identified regardless of incumbents or social norms (this is a requirement, since positions are used to define norms). For example, the positions in the sector of family social structure are given by universal kinship terms (e.g., Schusky, 1965). The position of "husband" is defined as a point that satisfies the condition of "a married male." Note that this position may be found for any particular society, regardless of the differing definitions and practices of marriage. The positions are contentless points (as in geometry) that receive meaning in relation to acts and the associated modalities. Any act may be related to a position by the modalities of whether the act is *permitted* to that position, *required* of that position, or *forbidden* for that position. (Merton, 1949, identifies four modalities: prescription, preference, permission, and proscription.) This relation between an act (e.g., washing dishes), a position (e.g., husband), and a modality (e.g., permitted) represents a social norm or rule for a given culture or social system. (Note the parallel in this meaning of "norm" with the commonly agreed-upon rules in chess: A chess piece's actions are permitted, required, or forbidden according to its position both on the board and in the hierarchy of pieces. Furthermore, the rules of chess are established by strong conventions, and transgressors are sanctioned as cheaters. For further elaboration see Chapters 8, 9, and 10.)

The institution of the family is constructed of the social norms regarding the acts that are permitted, forbidden, or required for positions in the kinship/family social structure. Norms are the basic building blocks of roles and role relationships. For example, a role is composed of all the activities permitted, required, or forbidden to a given position. Thus, there is often confusion between the analytic point of a position in a kinship chart and a social role when both are called "husband." For example, a relationship between two roles is defined by the sector of activities proscribed and prescribed for both roles. Thus, it may be permitted for husbands to commit adultery and forbidden for wives to do the same, but this makes little difference to the fact that this is an area in which roles (or, more precisely, norms for these positions) intersect regarding the activity of adultery.

So far, it seems that the institution of the family is being characterized in a static way, similar to the efforts of previous theorists. The connection with dynamic analysis does not come about by adding the dimension of time to static concepts, but, rather, by examining how norms and roles define stages of development. Aldous (1978) offers the following definition of "stage":

> A stage is a division within the lifetime of a family that is distinctive enough from those that precede and follow it to constitute a separate period. It presupposes qualitative changes so readily discernible that earlier interaction patterns cluster together in clear distinction from later phenomena. (p. 80)

The concept of "stage" is a familiar one in the study of both individual and family development. The fact that a stage of family development is supposed to be marked by interaction patterns that are qualitatively distinct from previous and subsequent interaction patterns suggests that the norms governing these interaction patterns (role relationships) must be different as well. Thus, the concept of stages in family development stands for periods of time in which there are relatively homogeneous norms and roles, as opposed to the heterogeneity between periods of time standing for different stages.

It may seem that the view that institutional timing and sequencing norms govern family stage transitions is a deterministic perspective. However, that is far from the case. In the theory of family development, it is recognized that even at the institutional level, sequencing and timing norms for individuals and families do not just originate within the institution of the family. They also come from within other institutions such as education, as well as from the norms synchronizing the timing of events between institutions. This implies that the trajectory or path that a family may follow, based on family institutional norms, is only a probable one. The process of family transitions for families and individuals is a stochastic process, in which not all of the many factors that affect the transition from stage to stage are known, nor can they necessarily be specified.

The concept of stages of family development has been problematic for theorists. For instance, Aldous (1978, pp. 83–93) discusses at least five different ways of demarcating stages in family development. Borne et al. (1979) have pointed out that the various conceptualizations of stages fail to include relevant stage categories for single-parent families, childless marriages, remarried families, and many other family forms. The logical constraints on a stage conception are (1) that it should be exhaustive of all the possible stages of family development, and (2) that it should be impossible for any two stages to occur simultaneously. These constraints (exhaustiveness and mutual exclusivity) have proved difficult ones for theorists. For example, the Duvall and Hill (1948) stages include "families with preschool children" and "families with school children." Clearly, some families may have both preschool and school-age children. Regardless of which stages are used, the requirements of exclusivity and exhaustiveness continue to be problems for theorists to solve.

One way to resolve this problem is to pursue some implications inherent in the theoretical notion of stages of development. Since stages are supposed to be qualitatively distinct periods, it seems that the changes between stages, by implication, are disjunctive in character. Another way of saying this is that a new stage must represent a noticeable disjunction with the preceding stage. This is a clear implication entailed in the definition of "stage." The point of transition is called an "event." Allison (1984) defines an event as follows:

> [A]n event consists of some qualitative change that occurs at a specific point in time. One would not ordinarily use the term "event" to describe a gradual change in some quantitative variable. The change must consist of a relatively sharp disjunction between what precedes and what follows. (p. 9)

This definition of "event" clearly has many similarities to the definition of "stage." The similarities suggest that events are the transition points between stages. This addition further suggests a way to avoid some of the difficulties with the specification of stages that are both exclusive and exhaustive. An event either occurs or does not occur at some specific time point or within a particular time interval. For this reason, event analysis can provide categories that are both exhaustive and exclusive.

To sum up this discussion, norms construct relatively unique and homogeneous periods in family life (stages), bounded by family transition events. As mentioned earlier in this discussion, the concept of the family career offers a dynamic rather than a static conception of family organization. The concept of a career, whether family or individual, entails a sequence of events (or stages) over time. This sequence of transition events may be developmental if the probability of an event is determined by the duration of time since the previous event. The alternative way of stating this is the following: The sequence of stages is a developmental process *if* the probability of being in a stage is dependent upon the duration of the previous stage. Thus, *family development is the process whereby stages of family life are sequenced so that the probability of any stage is determined by the duration of time in a specific previous stage.*

EVENT SEQUENCING AND TIMING

An event is not just an operational way of dealing with stages. Rather, the concepts of stage and event are intimately related, in much the same way as a line and a point are related in geometry. In general, it is the responsibility of researchers to identify both the stage and the events associated with its beginning and end. However, it should be noted that a stage is a necessary condition for there being an event, but the reverse is not necessarily true. Not all events are family transition events; there are historical events or occurrences that may not mark a stage transition. However, a family stage necessarily implies at least one family transition event. In this book, the term "event" is reserved solely for transition events and not for any other occurrences. This use of the term is most consistent with the definition by Allison (1984), given above.

An event marks both the end of the preceding stage and the beginning of the subsequent stage. For example, the birth of a child marks the end of the marital dyad stage and the beginning of the early family stage. However, most people who have experienced this transition know only too well that the exact date of the birth event fails to convey the nature of the transition as they have experienced it. For instance, attending prenatal classes, the pregnancy, taking out life insurance, and equipping the nursery usually occur some months before the date of birth. Yet these experiences are associated more with the early family than they are with the marital dyad. This has led some scholars to propose that continuous changes accumulate to the point at which new norms apply (Rodgers, 1973). Other scholars, such as Pearlin and Schooler (1978), conceptualize this as "anticipatory socialization." This raises two critical issues for the theory: the validity of events as points, and the relationship between continuous and discrete change. The latter issue is addressed first.

The relationship between continuous and discrete change is quite clear once we identify what is changing and in regard to which level of analysis. Most of an individual's experience may seem to be a continuous flow of occurrences. However, the theory of family development is not a phenomenological theory that attempts to explain an individual's perception of his or her experience; rather, the theory focuses on the transitions of family stages. Since family stages are defined by the institutional norms, the unit that changes discretely is a set of norms. Although an expectant married couple may experience anticipatory socialization for the next stage, the set of expectations does not change until the child is born and the spouses become parents. They may practice roles, but this is nothing but "play" until the child arrives. If there is a miscarriage, then it becomes even more clear that such role practice is identical to the anticipatory socialization that children go through when playing "doctor." Thus, normative sets change in a discrete and disjunctive way, even though individual experience may seem more continuous. In general, then, continuous change of social norms goes on all the time within an institution, but the stages that are defined as sets of norms appropriate to a particular form of social group are discrete.

The issue of the validity of events as transition points also becomes clearer when the levels of analysis are separated. Clearly, events can be valid indicators of stages when stages are the sets of norms appropriate to a particular family group structure. For example, the birth of the first child clearly distinguishes the marital dyad from the early family, since one group has only two affinally related adults and the other group has two affinally related adults and a consanguineally related offspring. The structures are different, and there are different normative sets for each structure. Thus, events are valid as transition points when they clearly demarcate changes in group structure *and* there are distinct sets of institutional norms for the different group structures.

The sequencing of stages necessarily implies the sequencing of events. The sequencing of events contains three dimensions: the events themselves, the order of events, and the timing of events. These are the three essential dimensions necessary for studying a developmental career. An event does not just represent a demarcation between stages; it undoubtedly has an influence of its own on subsequent events. The sequence of events contains the individual influences of many events, as well as the influence of the particular order of the events. For example, the events of first marriage, first child, and first divorce for an individual can have quite different effects, depending on whether the order for these events is (1) marriage, child, and divorce or (2) child, marriage, and divorce. And, to establish whether a process is developmental, the timing of the events in a sequence is essential.

There are at least three aspects to the timing of a single event, such as the birth of a first child. We can discuss timing in terms of (1) the *age* of one individual, such as the mother; (2) the *duration* of the dyad, such as length of marriage; or (3) the chronological *date,* which would also indicate period effects.

For event sequences, in which at least two events are used and one event precedes the other, timing of events can be discussed in terms of (1) the *duration* of time between events, which would also give the duration of the stage; (2) the *target individual's age* when each event occurred; (3) the *family's age* when each event occurred, which might be measured by length of marriage, time since birth of the first child, or the like; or (4) the chronological *date* at which each event occurred.

It may be that some sequences are series of event transitions, in which duration dependence begins at some point other than birth (e.g., marriage). Alternatively, it may be that some sequences are series of age-graded transitions, in which duration dependence is tied to chronological or birth age of the individual or family. (Both types of transitions and duration dependences are discussed in "Change and Development," above.) It is often the case that the two types of duration dependences are empirically present and cannot be disentangled. This issue is discussed more fully in Chapter 5.

CONCLUSION: LEVELS OF FAMILY CAREER ANALYSIS

In this concluding section, I return to the notion of levels of analysis as a way to summarize and describe how the theoretical concepts are used at each level. More precisely, a return to the topic of levels of analysis accomplishes two goals. First, since each level of analysis may contain several units of analysis, a return to each level is necessary to add specificity to the theory. Second, because each level of analysis requires a somewhat different treatment as to family development, there is a need to clarify this variation in treatment. However, the concepts of family development, stage, event, sequence of events, and timing of events are common to all levels of analysis.

The fifth level of analysis is that of the institution of the family. At this level, the construct to be analyzed is the social norm. Social norms govern family activities at all levels. There are two major types of social norms to be analyzed at this level, as Hogan (1978) points out: (1) the norms that govern the sequencing and timing of family events, and (2) the norms that coordinate the timing and sequencing of family norms with the timing and sequencing of norms for other social institutions, such as politics, religion, work, and education. Although this interinstitutional level of analysis can be viewed as a separate level above the institution of the family, the unit of analysis remains that of the norms about events, their sequencing, and their timing.

Aldous (1978) draws a graphic picture of the need for coordination among the norms of these various social institutions. Clearly, if all of these social institutions have stage- and age-graded norms such that when an individual is a certain age he or she is expected to get married, have a child, finish school, start a first job, move into a house, buy a car, purchase furniture, and experience the deaths of parents, the stress resulting from all of these social expectations would be devastating. Rather, social institutions are so organized as to synchronize the various age-graded norms among institutions; in other words, there are cross-institutional norms regarding the sequencing and timing of events among institutions. Thus, both norms within the institution and those between institutions can be analyzed.

The fourth level of analysis is the level of populations of families. At this level, families as an aggregate show variability in sequences and timing for events. This level of analysis studies the distribution of sequences and the variation in timing. The concepts added at this level of analysis are conformity to and deviance from the social norms. Clearly, the greater the conformity to a social norm regarding the timing or sequencing of family events, the stronger the consensus regarding these norms. Deviance from the normative family career is thus a statistical property belonging to aggregated families. To explain deviance from a family career sequence, other aggregate characteristics, such as age cohort, historical period, or social class groupings, may be used to detect homogeneous clusters within these categories.

The third level of analysis is that of a family. The analysis of family development for a particular family is sequential. The ideas of conformity to and deviance from the social norms are also useful at this level of analysis. The career of a family can only be studied sequentially or retrospectively. Again, the principal constructs are the events themselves, the timing of events, the duration between events, and the sequencing of events.

The second level is that of the family's subunits. These subunits are the role relationships constructed and defined by social norms. As at all other levels, development is analyzed in terms of events, the sequence of events and their timing. At this level, the role relationships are what develop over time. For example, the core role relationship in the family is that of parent and child. This role relationship goes through various transitions, some of which are age-graded and some of which are event-graded. The events for the many different units or role relationships, such as parent–child, sibling, marital, and grandparental, are likely to have some developmental commonalities as well as some uniqueness, based on the differences in the norms constructing these role relationships.

The last level of analysis is the individual level. At first it may seem that individuals do little other than compose the role relationships in the family. However, the individual is the unit of analysis that *experiences* the family career as his or her family career or family history. So even though there may be several members of the same family, their family histories are distinctly different. For example, some of the events such as the birth of the first child are experienced by different people at different ages and not experienced at all by subsequent siblings. The family career of the individual is not the family's career, but nonetheless may be analyzed by the constructs of events, their sequences, and their timing. Furthermore, an individual's family career can be analyzed as to its conformity to or deviance from the aggregate of individuals' sequencing and timing of events. An important point in regard to the individual unit of analysis is that individual development is not of direct interest or concern. The theory of family development deals with *family* at each level of analysis. At the individual level, the focus is on family development as experienced by the individual, as one of five facets reflecting family development.

The concepts introduced thus far represent the starting point for a truly dynamic characterization of the family. However, it remains a crucial task for the theory to specify the ramifications implicit in the definition of family development. It is with this objective in mind that I now turn to the formal modeling of the theory.

CHAPTER 4

The Process of Development: Substantive Theory and Model

Chapter 3 has introduced many of the basic concepts and perspectives of the theory of family development. This chapter elaborates those concepts that are important in the specification of the *process of development*. When the theory of family development is compared to other family theories, the one feature highlighted is that the theory of family development is directly concerned with the specification of a process. This chapter focuses on the exact nature of this process.

Although several theorists have discussed the developmental process (e.g., Magrabi & Marshall, 1965; Rodgers, 1973; Hill & Mattessich, 1979; Mattessich & Hill, 1987), it has remained a somewhat loosely defined notion in regard to changes in the family. The approach taken here is first to identify the general way in which previous scholars have discussed the process of family development. The definition of "development" by Featherman (1985) is compared to other definitions. The strengths of Featherman's definition are that (1) it makes it possible to distinguish all family change from developmental change; (2) it suggests an exact mathematical model for the process; and (3) it largely encompasses other scholars' understanding of the process.

The theory of family development and the model of the process of development must be compatible. That is, the assumptions of the theory should *fit* with the assumptions of the model. As noted in Chapter 2, Leik and Meeker (1975) characterize this task as the formalization of theory. When a theory is mapped onto a model, it is said to be formalized. This process of formalization interprets the substantive propositions of the theory more precisely as a set of symbols and relations among those symbols. This process often weeds out contradictions and requires that the theorist make choices in order to resolve any ambiguities in the theory. Thus, the process of formalization may systematize and clarify the theory. Once the model is specified, the mathematical properties of the model may be interpreted substantively, sometimes yielding new insights into the substantive theory or generating new substantive propositions.

This chapter forms the basic framework of a theory of family development. In Chapter 3, many of the basic concepts have been introduced and discussed; in this chapter, these concepts appear in the basic assumptions of the substantive theory. These substantive theoretical assumptions are mapped onto a mathematical model that serves as an analogue to the process of development that the theory identifies. Thus, this chapter explores the substantive theory, the model, and the relations between the theory and the model.

THEORETICAL OVERVIEW

The theory of family development has had many formulations since its inception in the work of Duvall and Hill (1948). Duvall (1971) used this approach in her text, the first edition of which was published in the 1950s. However, at this point the theory was largely a description of the way in which middle-class American families progressed from marriage to the postparental years. As such, it was specific to one particular historical period, 1940–1960, and it offered few if any universal theoretical propositions. It was in the work of Reuben Hill and his colleagues that the theory of family development began to take shape. Hill and Hansen (1960) identified the "developmental approach" as one of the major conceptual frameworks for the study of the family. Hill and Rodgers (1964) laid the foundation for later work by developing the notions of role relationships and their changes over time. This effort was further refined in the subsequent work by Rodgers (1973), who also defined the concepts of family career and the levels of analysis for the study of the family. The concept of the family career was even more thoroughly discussed by Aldous (1978). Aldous (1978) contributed the notions of family subsystem careers and the idea that the timing of the family career must be coordinated with that of the individual's other careers, such as work and educational careers. Most recently, Mattessich and Hill (1987) have described all of the various strands of theoretical work associated with developmental theory, including stress theory.

If one were to identify one theoretical notion that characterizes the theory of family development for most academics, it would be the idea of the "family life cycle" (Glick, 1947). This idea conjures up the picture of the family as an organism having a life cycle, just as the individual members of the family do. However, the notion of "life cycle" has undergone significant changes in areas devoted to the study of individuals, such as developmental psychology, where the term "life course" is now preferred. A similar re-evaluation has occurred in the theory of family development. Critics such as Feldman and Feldman (1975) argued that family development was neither cyclical nor entirely analogous to the ways in which individuals develop. However, Rodgers (1973) had already substituted the concept of the "family career." Aldous (1978) obviously endorsed this move by entitling her book *Family Careers*.

The family career, previously discussed in Chapter 3, is defined as the sequence of configurations of role relationships over the family's life as a group. Several elements of this definition must be clarified. First, the idea of a sequence can include both the process (sequencing) and the result (the sequence as history). The concept of the family career contains both of these meanings—process and product of the process. It is important, however, for a theory of family development to emphasize the process rather than the resulting family history. It is crucial that the theory be concerned with the process, since an understanding of the process will contain and predict the history. So, even though family development deals with the history of families, that history is a product of the *process* of family development.

A second element contained in the concept of the family career is that role relationships in the family are linked sequentially over time. This implies that the role relationships are linked as either *continuous* or *discrete* changes over time. On this point there is considerable agreement. Almost all developmental theorists have accepted the notion that there are discrete stages in the developmental process. However, it would be mistaken to say that there exists complete unanimity on this. For example, Rodgers (1973, pp. 48–49) states that many disjunctive changes are, upon deeper examination, really continuous in nature. And Mattessich and Hill (1987, p. 444) discuss continuous versus discontinuous change as an unresolved issue for the model of family development. On the other hand, most developmentalists argue that the events marking stage transitions, such as the birth of a child or death of a spouse, are indicative of discrete and disjunctive stages rather than continuous ones. As previously argued in Chapter 3, individuals' experience around these events often appears continuous because of anticipatory socialization. However, when an event fails to occur the transition does not take place, no matter how much anticipatory socialization has taken place. Thus, the second point regarding the family career is that it is a process of transitions between discrete stages.

The disjunctive nature of stages may seem not entirely consistent with the definition of the family career as changing patterns of role relationships in the family. The seeming inconsistency lies in the fact that changes in role relationships can be either gradual and continuous or disjunctive and discrete. Clearly, then, there is some continuous change *within* stages; however, changes between stages are by definition disjunctive, discrete, and marked by an "event" (e.g., the birth of a first child marks the transition to roles of parenthood). This distinction is also made by Mattessich and Hill (1987): "[W]ithin each stage, some growth also tends to occur (not enough to tip the scales and provoke reorganization) that is essentially continuous and quantitative" (p. 444).

The third element contained in the concept of the family career is that of time. The sequencing of stages implies that time is involved in this process. However, there seems to be some confusion in regard to the concept of time that is most appropriate to the theory of family development. For instance, Rodgers (1973) delineates three distinct notions of time useful in the study of development: "historical time," "social process time," and "chronological time." This last, "chronological time," is the most familiar to us, since it refers to the mechanical conception of time that we face every day on wristwatches and calendars. This mechanical notion of time is based on the periodicity of some physical phenomenon, such as water dripping in a water clock or a gear turning in a wristwatch. By "social process time," Rodgers means the qualitative and discrete nature of time as it is experienced. Thus, a certain stage of one's life may have qualitative characteristics that separate this period from others. For example, one might refer to "the time when I was divorced" or "the time when the kids were living at home" as distinctive periods in life. The idea of social process time is a phenomenological way of viewing time—time as experienced by the individual, dyad, or family (Borne et al., 1979). The last conception of time is what Rodgers calls "historical time." Here Rodgers means the effects of historical events, such as the Great Depression and the Vietnam war, on individuals and families. This type of time deals with the effects of these events and is currently examined in terms of period effects and the interaction of period and cohort effects. As such, historical time is not so much a conception of time as an identification of age and historical factors as they affect families and individuals.

The conceptions of chronological time and social process time are very important to a theory of family development, because they highlight a critical distinction between time and process. It is clear from Rodgers's discussion of social process time that he is trying to get at the notion that for a family the process of development proceeds and is experienced as distinct qualitative periods. The conception of chronological time is continuous and incremental rather than discrete. These two notions are not incompatible, but do get at different aspects of the phenomenon. For example, chronological time is useful when discussing age effects and comparing timing of events between families. On the other hand, social process time is useful in identifying periods of life as they are experienced by families. Of course, these two are not contradictory, and we can always examine how long (chronological time) a certain period (social process time) lasted for a family or individual. This distinction comes up again in the discussion of the incorporation of time in the model.

To sum up this discussion, the family career is composed of discrete stages; it is a process whereby families move from one stage to another in disjunctive transitions. The markers between these transitions are called "events" because of the disjunctive nature of these transition points. There is also a common pattern to the development of families because of the institutional norms regulating family development. As we shall see later, the theory of family development gains its nomothetic content from its view of institutional norms and the ways in which these norms guide and direct the family career.

DIMENSIONS OF PROCESSES

Before examining definitions of development, it is helpful to discuss some general notions about process. Several dimensions apply to the description of any process. The most basic dimension is whether the process is a "deterministic" or a "stochastic" process. A deterministic process is one in which a given state *necessarily* follows from certain conditions or preceding states. On the other hand, a stochastic process is one in which a given state only has a *probability* of following certain conditions or antecedent states. A deterministic process is naturally attached to the notion of causality. Indeed, the only reason we may not be able to predict a deterministic process accurately is that we have not measured or specified all of the relevant variables. The stochastic process is one for which, even if all factors were known, the outcome would still only be probable.

Another important dimension in describing any process, and one that has been discussed to some extent above, is whether the process is continuous or discrete in time. That is, does the process move only in discrete units of time or can it move continuously? For example, the budgets for most institutions change by discrete units of time, usually the fiscal year. On the other hand, having a second child may occur at any time, even though some time periods are more probable than others.

The last general dimension useful in characterizing a process is whether the units of the process vary in magnitude (quantitatively) or vary in type (qualitatively). The more usual way of stating this is to characterize the process as either a "continuous-variable" system or a "discrete-state" system. These should not be confused with the distinction made above in regard to time. The distinction regarding the type of system simply tells us whether the unit of analysis varies as levels of a continuous variable or as states. The term "state" refers to a qualitative unit that is part of a set, which is exhaustive of all the possible states a system may occupy. For example, if we suppose that families can be in only one of the states of growth, shrinkage, or stability, and that there are no other possible states in this system (exhaustive), then this is a discrete-state system.

These three dimensions can be used to characterize any particular process. They are especially useful in making clear the exact nature of the process of family development. But first, it is important to define what we mean by "family development."

DEFINITION OF FAMILY DEVELOPMENT

Aldous (1978), like other theorists before her, approaches the process of development by way of the concept of "developmental tasks." She characterizes the process as being what she labels a series of "limited linkages" (Aldous, 1978, p. 110). A "limited linkage" refers to a situation in which a stage is only in part determined by the preceding stage. Aldous states that "The level the family attains in task performance depends in part on the demands of the new stage, in part on the continuing effects of past performance" (1978, p. 110). In order to clarify this relationship, Aldous cites the "game-tree model" developed by Magrabi and Marshall (1965). Basically, the game-tree model is a branching process. An example of such a process is useful. Imagine that a system has three states, a, b, and c. Furthermore, imagine that for this system time moves in discrete units. For simplicity, suppose that the probabilities for a, b, and c are equal, .33. Then the process could be diagrammed as the branching process shown in Figure 4.1.

The important point regarding Aldous's use of the term "limited

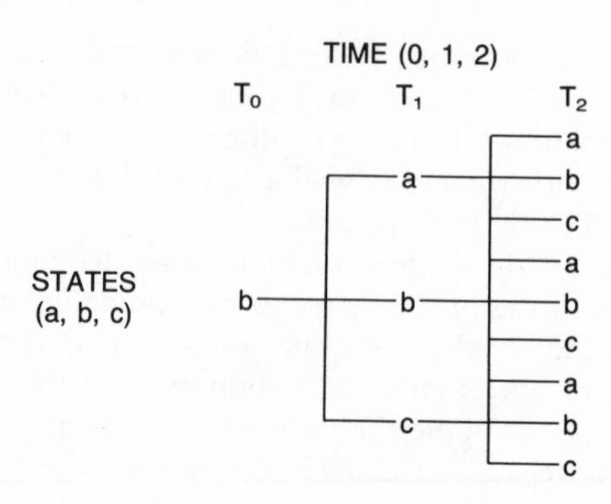

FIGURE 4.1. Example of a game-tree diagram.

linkage," her citation of the Magrabi and Marshall (1965) model, and the fact that the Magrabi and Marshall model is a probabilistic branching process is that development is characterized as a stochastic rather than a deterministic system. So even though Aldous (1978) does not directly define a developmental process, she nonetheless characterizes it as a stochastic process.

Hill and Mattessich (1979) developed a working definition of family development:

> Family development refers to the process of progressive structural differentiation and transformation over the family's history, to the active acquisition and selective discarding of roles by incumbents of family positions as they seek to meet the changing functional requisites for survival and as they adapt to recurring life stresses as a family system. (1979, p. 174)

This is a complex definition of the process; however, Mattessich and Hill (1987) state that it contains three aspects crucial to understanding the process. First, family development is both an organizational and an interactional phenomenon. Second, there is a continuity of behavior in families over time. And third, there are two sources of change: functional requirements and life stresses.

Nevertheless, this definition fails to clarify the process in several ways. First, it does not address the characteristics of a process, such as continuous versus discrete time, variable versus state system, and deterministic versus stochastic nature of the process. In this regard, it does not even go as far as the Aldous (1978) discussion. Second, it fails to help us understand "how" the process moves through time, other than saying that it is "progressive." Third, it seems to suggest a causal relationship between changes in family stage on the one hand and functional requirements and life stresses on the other. This is confusing, not only because the literature does not support this perspective, but also because it is contrary to the part of the definition stating that the process is one of "structural differentiation." It is difficult for a family scholar to believe that people have children (structural differentiation) because of functional requirements and/or life stresses.

One major problem in defining family development is distinguishing development from other forms of change in families. Featherman (1985) suggests,

> The special feature which discriminates development from such generic quantitative and qualitative change in time is *duration dependence,* a characteristic of the rate of change. If the rate of leaving (or entering) a state is a function of the time spent in that state, then change is dependent upon duration. (p. 215)

The idea of "duration dependence" seems to fit well with the notion that family development is the process by which families change from one stage to another. It adds the element that the probability of moving from one stage to another is based on the duration of time spent in the previous stage. This probability may not be a monotonic function; it can be curvilinear.

If Featherman's definition is adapted for the particular process of family development, the resulting definition would be as follows: *Family development is a process in which families move from stage to stage and the probability of a transition from one stage* (i) *to another stage* (j) *is dependent on the duration of time in the previous stage* (i).

This definition has several strengths that the previous definition by Hill and Mattessich (1979) does not have. These strengths are that (1) it makes it possible to distinguish all family change from developmental change; (2) it suggests an exact mathematical model for the process; and (3) it largely encompasses other scholars' understanding of the process.

This definition does share some common elements with the Hill and Mattessich (1979) definition, as well as the understanding most scholars have regarding development. For example, the proposed definition includes the aspect of "structural differentiation" discussed by Hill and

Mattessich—that is, the view of stages as distinct structural units. A transition from one state to another, then, would encompass the idea of structural differentiation. However, the notion that the process is "progressive," or directed in some teleological way, would not be viable in the proposed definition of development. Also, the proposed definition is consistent with the meaning of development in other areas of social science, especially individual life span development.

Borne et al. (1979) suggested that the process of development can follow any of three models: a discrete-stage process, a process based on transition periods, or a continuous dynamic process. Although these authors did not specify that the process is not deterministic, this is implied by their models. These models are not mutually exclusive. Indeed, the definition of development offered above contains all three of these models. The definition of development used here incorporates the concept of stages as discrete entities; the concept of a transition period as dependent upon the duration of a stage; and the idea of the continuous transition rate from one stage to another as a continuous dynamic process. The exact way in which each of the elements suggested by Borne et al. is incorporated becomes clearer when the theoretical model is discussed. However, the present definition of family development does incorporate each of these and is largely consistent with the way in which scholars such as Borne et al. have discussed family development as a process.

The proposed definition of family development makes it possible to distinguish developmental change from other types of change in families. Sometimes developmental change has been confused with other types of family processes and change. One consequence of this confusion has been that the theory of family development has then been expected to explain all change in families, rather than limited to the more appropriate task of explaining developmental change in families. Some of the other types of change in families are random change and adaptive change. These are more fully discussed in Chapter 7.

The greatest strength of the proposed definition is that it helps us to specify a precise model for the process of family development. Not only does such a model reduce the vagueness and consequent confusion associated with imprecise definitions, but it also helps clarify the substantive meaning of the theory. The remainder of this chapter is devoted to this topic.

In order to address the theoretical significance of this definition, I now turn to a discussion of the relationship among the assumptions and propositions of the theory, the model they imply, and this definition of family development.

THEORETICAL ASSUMPTIONS AND PROPOSITIONS

It is the purpose of this section to introduce a few assumptions and propositions from the theory of family development for the purpose of developing a model of the process of family development. The points presented here are those that have been identified as central to the theory (Aldous, 1978).

The theory of family development characterizes family activity as regulated by institutional norms. These norms regulate which events are permitted, required, and forbidden; the order in which families should sequence stages; and the duration of those stages. The role relationships within the family are also governed by these institutional norms, since roles and role relationships are composed of norms. Individual maturation and capacity, whether fast or slow, has little to do with the normative structure. For example, we regard the moron and the genius with much the same reaction: Both are deviant.

"Family development" refers to the process by which families make transitions to different stages. These stages are defined by the institutional norms. What goes on within a stage is defined by the norms composing the role relationships in the family. The relationship between stages is defined by the events that signify the beginning and end of a stage. The temporal structure is defined by the sequence and timing norms for stages or events. The process of family development means different things for different units of analysis. For the individual, development is experienced as distinct periods of family life, such as "when we were a young married couple" or "when the kids were small." Not only are these stages experienced as qualitatively discrete periods by the members of the family; much more importantly, they are defined as periods by the larger normative system. So, for example, a couple may experience the addition of a child as a joyous start to a new period in their lives, while the institutional norms prescribe that the new roles of father and mother be added to husband and wife. At the aggregate level of families, stages are a construct of the uniformity of institutional norms governing the sequencing and timing of events.

This picture of family development has been shared by many authors. For example, Aldous (1978) characterizes the theory of family development in terms of the following assumptions:

1. Family behavior is the sum of past experience of family members as incorporated in the present as well as in their goals and expectations for the future.
2. Families develop and change over time in similar and consistent ways.

3. Humans not only initiate actions as they mature and interact with others but also they react to environmental pressures.
4. The family and its members must perform certain time-specific tasks set by themselves and by persons in the broader society.
5. In a social setting, the individual is the basic autonomous unit. (p. 15)

These assumptions are largely in agreement with the perspective taken here. For example, the first one asserts that at the individual level of analysis, family history has an effect on behavior leading to future states. The second assumption implies that *families* make the transitions between states in relatively consistent patterns. When this second assumption is linked to the fourth one, the picture emerges that families' sequencing and timing are consistent because of the normative system. The third and fifth assumptions state that the internal structure of stages is relatively similar; if this is coupled with the fourth assumption, we find that this consistency is a result of the normative structure.

There are, however, some distinct differences. First, the fifth assumption appears to view the individual as a distinctly important level of analysis. This is what Featherman (1985) has called "personological thinking" and is certainly different from the approach taken here. By contrast, the approach here is that institutional norms construct the behavior of families, a family, role relationships, and the individual's experience of the family. The emphasis on the individual might be more appropriate in a theory of individual development than in a theory of family development.

Another difference is that the second assumption seems to imply that change and development are roughly the same. In Chapter 3, great care has been taken to draw the distinction between these terms. That discussion specifies that development is a particular form of change defined by the duration dependence of stages.

Yet another difference is the interpretation of the fourth assumption: "The family and its members must perform certain time-specific tasks *set by themselves* and *by persons in the broader society*" (italics added). The notion of "developmental tasks" (Havighurst, 1948) seems redundant with the concept of "norms." Norms establish expectations that are internalized by individuals, but, much more importantly, these norms compose the social institutions of any social system. Norms are not "set" by individuals, but are only expressed by individuals, as in the statement "This is a good time to have children." Thus, the notion of developmental tasks seems to confuse levels of analysis and to conceal the point that the developmental theory of the family is not a theory about individual development.

If the areas of disagreement and vagueness are removed from the assumptions above, the core assumptions of the theory become clear and relatively precise. Relying on the foregoing discussion of the assumptions listed by Aldous (1978), as well as the discussion in Chapter 3, we find the following assumptions, definitions, and propositions:

1. Development is a process in which the probability of a new stage depends on the duration of time in the present stage (Featherman, 1985). {def.}
2. Stages are qualitatively distinct periods of experience for individuals, of role relationships for family subunits, of expectations for a family, and of modal behavior for families. {def.}
3. A stage is bounded by events at the beginning and end of the period, so that events represent transition points. {ass.}
4. The sequence of events or stages is called the family career. {def.}
5. Previous stages influence present stages. {prop.}
6. The order of stages for a family is not invariant or irreversible. {ass.}
7. Families develop in consistent patterns over time. {prop.}
8. Family development is a relatively consistent process because it is governed by stage-graded and timing (duration and sequencing) institutional norms. {prop.}
9. Norms both from other social institutions and between social institutions affect the timing and sequencing of events in the family. {prop.}

An examination of these nine points suggests the characteristics of the process of development. Since the process is reversible (6), it is clearly not a monotonic, nonrecursive linear model, but a continuous-time model (6, 8). Since the process is based on probabilities attributed not simply to measurement error but to the process itself (1), it is a stochastic process. Points 2 and 3 indicate that the process is composed of discrete states or events. The process of development, then, seems to be a discrete-state, continuous-time, stochastic process.

A MODEL OF DEVELOPMENT

The model proposed here may be familiar to some developmental theorists. The application of such a model to family development was first suggested in the work of Magrabi and Marshall (1965). They proposed a game-tree model of family development in which the nodes of the "tree" represented transitions to other stages in the process. Rodgers (1973) suggested that Markov chains might prove a useful way in which to analyze family development. More recently, a colleague and I (White & Reid, 1984) applied a discrete-time, discrete-state Markov model to family development. All of this work suggests the appropriateness of some form of Markov process as a model for the process of family development. However, the case for the "fit" between the model and the substantive points of the theory necessitates a detailed examination of the model.

The model proposed here is familiar to sociologists as a continuous-time, discrete-state semi-Markov model. This model was first introduced to sociologists by Coleman (1964); more recent formulations in sociology are found in the works by Coleman (1981) and Tuma and Hannan (1984). The continuous-time, discrete-state model has not received the attention and empirical application that the more popular discrete-time, discrete-state model has received. As Tuma and Hannan (1984) point out, the semi-Markov model is a general model "which includes binomial and multinomial models, renewal models, discrete time Markov models, and time-stationary Markov models as special cases" (p. 96). Thus, the more popular discrete-time model may be seen as a restricted version of the more general model.

The reason most often cited for using the continuous-time model rather than the discrete-time model is that it is more realistic. The discrete-time model assumes equal time intervals between "steps" or transitions in the process. It seems clear that few events are experienced with such exact periodicity. For example, we cannot expect the time intervals from first date to marriage, from marriage to the birth of the first child, and from birth of the first child to birth of the second child to be the same interval for any one person, let alone for most people. It seems more accurate to model the process in terms of continuous change from one state to another. Not only does this seem a more accurate representation of most people's experience; it also appears to be a more accurate reflection of the substantive theory of family development.

The first substantive point listed above is that the probability of a new stage depends on the duration of time in the present stage. This idea of duration dependence suggests that a continuous-time process is more appropriate for two reasons. First, clearly, the *duration* of time in a state is a continuous rather than a discrete notion. Second, even though it is possible to model a continuous process with a discrete-time model, such a model would assume that length of time in a state is monotonically related to the probability of a transition to some other state. In many situations, we can see that this assumption is terribly inaccurate. One example is that of the probability of having a first child, given that the present state is a marriage. At first the probability of having a child increases with time married, but at some point this is reversed: The longer the duration of the marriage without children, the *less* the probability that any children will be born to that marriage. This argument for a continuous-time model can only be fully appreciated as other aspects of the model are elaborated.

Before the discussion turns to the details of the model, a general overview is needed. This overview is especially oriented toward scholars who find the mathematical terms unfamiliar. First, it is crucial to know that a "Markov model" is a model of process or changes. The basic construct of such a model is the "state." A state is one member of a set of qualitative categories that are mutually exclusive and exhaustive. The set of states represents all the possible states of the system, and any two states cannot be occupied simultaneously by the same individual (or unit of analysis). A matrix that has the complete set of states in identical order on the row and column dimensions is called a "transition matrix." The cells of such a matrix represent all of the possible transitions of the system from time 1 to time 2. For instance, imagine that a simple system of family development has only three states, growth, stability, and shrinkage (e.g., Rodgers, 1973, pp. 12–13). In this simplistic example, a family would be in the growth stage if it were adding members to the household, stable if it were neither adding nor subtracting members, and shrinking if it were losing members. Clearly, at time zero we could start with marriage as the beginning of the growth stage, followed by the addition of children as further steps in this growth stage. Then the middle years for most families would be the stage of stability, followed by children's leaving home and a spouse's death in the shrinkage stage. When we examine the family's development as a process, the focus is on the transitions of movements from being in one stage to being in another stage. If we followed 100 families through their lives as a group, we would find that not every one would follow the pattern described above in such a lockstep fashion. For various reasons unknown to us, some families would have infant deaths, others would have divorces and remarriages, and relatives would come to live with still others. The actual transition matrix might look something like the imaginary one in Table 4.1.

This simple discrete-time model serves to introduce the terms of "state," "transition probability," and "transition matrix" in a straightforward, nontechnical manner. In the imaginary transition matrix (Table 4.1), each cell contains the proportion of the sample in a given state at

TABLE 4.1. Transition Matrix for Three Imaginary States of Family Development

State at time 1	State at time 2		
	Growth	Stability	Shrinkage
Growth	.60	.30	.10
Stability	.10	.10	.80
Shrinkage	.05	.05	.90

time 1 that moved to another state at time 2. So, of those occupying the state "growth" at time 1, 60% were still in that state at time 2. According to these fictional data, once a family entered the "shrinkage" state, the probability of its staying in that state would be very high (.90).

This example is instructive when we return to the argument for the continuous-time, discrete-state semi-Markov model. Although many families would traverse their life course as a group in a stepwise pattern of growth followed by stability followed by shrinkage, some families might have a mother die in childbirth. A discrete-time model would appear contradictory in this case because the time frames for such a model are usually equal intervals of months or years, not minutes. But, for example, in a mother's death in childbirth, the child's birth and the mother's death may only be separated by minutes in time. A continuous-time model can handle such an occurrence in terms of either units of its time scale or fractions of units. Furthermore, we avoid another problem of the discrete-time model, which is that the apparent simultaneous occurrence of events suggests that the states are not mutually exclusive. From the perspective of the discrete-time model, it would appear in the example of the mother's death in childbirth that the growth state and the shrinkage state are simultaneous. This simultaneous occurrence violates the assumption that the states are mutually exclusive. This problem can be avoided with the continuous-time model.

The general model can be defined without mathematical notation. The model contains a given set of states of the system. At any one time, the system can be in only one of these states. The process moves from one state to another, and these moves are called "transitions." A transition from one state to another depends at most on the conditional probability, which is the probability of being in state X at time 2, given that the previous state was Y at time 1. Thus, an important constraint on the model is that the history for a family (or unit of analysis) is limited to this conditional probability or "transition probability." The continuous-time, discrete-state semi-Markov model depends on the duration of time for which the family was in the previous state. So this particular model gives more detailed consideration to the "transition rate" for families spending various lengths of time in a state. It is a characteristic of some particular systems that over time they reach an asymptote, or, rather, are stationary or equilibrium distributions. However, this is not a necessary characteristic of the model, but a derived characteristic of some particular parameterized models.

In more precise language, a continuous-time, discrete-state semi-Markov model is defined, following Coleman (1981), as a finite, countable set of states. Each individual (unit of analysis) has a probability of being in one specific state at time *t*. At time *t*, there is a transition rate between each pair of states *i* and *j*, $q_{ij}(t)$. This transition rate (q_{ij}) is given as the limit of the ratio of the transition probability, such that

$$q_{ij}(t) = \lim_{\Delta t \to 0} \frac{r_{ij}(t, t + \Delta t)}{\Delta t} \quad i \neq j \tag{1}$$

(Coleman, 1981, p. 9)

This defines the instantaneous transition rate from any state *i* to state *j*. Tuma and Hannan (1984) show that the an instantaneous transition rate may also be defined as the product of the hazard function and the conditional probability. More importantly, they point out that a semi-Markov process can make two assumptions regarding these transition rates. The transition rates may be expressed as dependent either on the duration of time in the last state or on the time of the last event. Because of mathematical difficulties in models dealing with both, Tuma and Hannan (1984, p. 95) suggest that the model be constrained to just duration dependence. The process is then defined by a system of differential equations represented, for example, by the following:

$$\frac{dp_i(t)}{dt} = -p_i \sum q_{ij}(t) + \sum_{j \neq i} p_j(t)\, q_{ji}(t) \tag{2}$$

(Coleman, 1981, p. 9)

For a excellent discussion of the relation between the transition probabilities of the discrete-time process and the instantaneous transition rates, readers should see Coleman (1964, pp. 127–130). Coleman (1981) is quick to point out that this is a general model and that more restricted versions of it are usually called for in data analysis. These more restricted models are discussed in subsequent chapters. However, the task of the present chapter is to specify a model for the substantive theory, and the general model is most robust in that regard.

CORRESPONDENCE BETWEEN THE MODEL AND THE THEORY

The best way to proceed in regard to judging the fit between the proposed model and the substantive theory is to examine how well the model incorporates each of the assumptions and propositions of the theory of family development. Point 1 is that the probability of moving to stage X depends on the duration in stage Y. As previously discussed, this point conforms nicely to the notion of duration dependence captured in the model and its instantaneous transition rates.

The second substantive point in the theory of family development is that stages are qualitatively distinct periods. The notion of "stages" in family development is very similar to the idea of "states" in the stochastic system. Both are qualitative categories that are defined as mutually exclusive and exhaustive. Undoubtedly, some earlier versions of stages of family development cited by Aldous (1978) have not been mutually exclusive, as in the previously discussed example of "families with preschool children" and "families with school-age children" (see Chapter 3). Also, Borne et al. (1979) have pointed out that many versions of family stages have not been exhaustive. For example, single parents and remarried families are often excluded from these stage categories by oversight. However, thus far, no one compelling set of theoretical stages of family development has been universally adopted by scholars. In fact, many theorists such as Rodgers (1973) feel that the choice of stages is up to the researcher, depending on the focus of his or her study. Whether or not this should be the case is not the point here. Rather, any proposed set of stages of family development should be mutually exclusive and exhaustive. There is an argument to be made that the theory of family development does not have to specify the stages of family development, but only the events hypothesized as transition points. This argument is more fully examined later. At this point in the evolution of the substantive theory, it seems clear that the correspondence between the notions of "stage" and "state" is close indeed.

The third point in the substantive theory is really a definition of "event" (Allison, 1984). The definition of an event becomes more important later when the restricted models of family development are discussed. The point of correspondence between the model and the theory in regard to events is that for the model, an event is a disrete point in time at which there is a transition between states of the system. This meaning in the model seems very close to the definition of an event previously given in Chapter 3. There, an event is defined as the point between stages where there is a qualitative difference between the stage before the event and the stage after the event.

The fourth point defines the family career as the sequence of events or stages. This again is a definition that corresponds to the transitions of any given family or individual over time. In terms of the model, the most probable life course for families would be given by the most probable stages (or events) for the model. If the system is a stationary system, the most probable transitions can be estimated from aggregate data.

The fifth point is that previous stages influence present stages. The Markov assumption is that the probability of being in the next state is at most dependent on the current state. If this theoretical proposition is interpreted to mean that *experience* over many different states affects the transition probability to the next state, rather than just the current state, then the theory and the model are disjunctive. However, a closer examination of such a claim is warranted. For instance, imagine two families in which the ages of corresponding family members are the same. One family has gone through the events of being married, having a child, having a spouse die, and remarriage. The other family has been married and has had a child. The first family has clearly experienced more events than the second family. However, the model assumes that the probability of a second child for these families is based on the fact that they are both currently in the same stage; that is, they both are in a stage composed of parents and one offspring. The alternative view would assume that because the histories are different, the probabilities are different. Many examples spring to mind, such as appreciation and depreciation; it is doubtful how well these represent family processes, however. It does seem plausible that the next stage is dependent on the time spent in the current stage, though there is no necessity to this argument. Tuma and Hannan (1984) sum up this discussion as follows:

> When transition rates depend on experience, future changes (which are governed by the transition rates) depend on past occupancy of particular states, and not just on the current state. Thus, stochastic processes governed by experience-dependent rates are not Markovian. (p. 195)

The fit between the fifth theoretical point and the Markov assumption of conditional probabilities pivots on the interpretation of the meaning of "previous stages." The model is consistent with the view that since the probability of moving to the next state is dependent on the current state, and that retrospectively the probability of the current state was dependent on the preceding state, and so on, the model does incorporate history. However, if one particular state determines a subsequent outcome regardless of whether it is immediately preceding, then the process is not Markovian. This assumption is critical for the clarity of the theory and for the fit between the theory and the model. This critical question regarding the appropriateness of the Markov assumption is examined in some detail in later chapters. For the present, it is assumed that the interpretation of the fifth theoretical proposition corresponds to the Markov assumption.

The sixth point is that the order of stages is not invariant or irreversible. This assumption is compatible with the stochastic model. Assumption 6 clearly asserts that the process is not a deterministic process. Nor does it make possible the assumption of a simple linear model that is called stochastic because of the addition of measurement error. Rather, assumption 6 states that the process itself is a probabilistic and perhaps a nonmonotonic process. This stochastic model fits well with this particular theoretical proposition.

Assumption 7 states that families develop in consistent patterns over time. This is consistent with a nondeterministic system. The model is consistent with this proposition in that the patterns of development emerge as transition probabilities, instantaneous transition rates, and the equilibrium or stationary state of the system. Furthermore, the model can test the notion of the *consistent* patterns as both the homogeneity of the process and a possible equilibrium point of the process. This proposition appears to correspond nicely to the model.

The eighth point is that family development is a relatively consistent process because it is governed by stage-graded and timing (duration) institutional norms. As noted in the list above, this is a theoretical *proposition* rather than an assumption. A proposition relates to variables that are assumed to have a specific relationship. The eighth proposition is a causal assertion indicating covariance over time of changes in the norms regulating family life and changes in the patterns of transition probabilities and transition rates. The stochastic model is a model aimed at states of a unit of analysis. That unit of analysis is interpreted in this work as the family. Proposition 8, however, brings the social institution of the family into the picture. This must be considered to be endogenous to the *assumptions* of the model. Rather, this proposition is a statement regarding *why* there are relatively consistent patterns, why these patterns change over time, and the expectation that there is systematic covariance.

This proposition, however, is not inconsistent with the model, but is simply a theoretical proposition of great breadth and explanatory power (see Chapters 7, 8, and 9).

The ninth and last point is also a theoretical proposition. This proposition is that norms both from other social institutions and between social institutions affect the timing and sequencing of events in the family. This proposition asserts that other social institutions, such as work and religion, have norms regulating activities that have an effect on the family. Furthermore, it posits a set of norms between institutions such as work and the family that regulate and synchronize the timing of events between both institutions. For example, one is supposed to get a job before marrying. The ninth proposition proposes a complex fabric of normative culture that is relatively consistent and homogeneous. These institutional norms and between institution norms must also be considered as exogenous to the model. Thus, these norms affect the process of family development but are exogenous to the model of family development. In this sense, the ninth proposition, like the eighth, is neither consistent nor inconsistent; rather, it implies a number of influences on family development that are examined in subsequent chapters.

EXPLANATIONS

As discussed in Chapter 2, a model does not supply an explanation in isolation from the substantive theory. Indeed, the model may specify the process and lead to the deduction of unforeseen theoretical implications, or it may improve the theory's predictive capacity, but it cannot explain an occurrence without being tied to the substantive theory. What would such an explanation look like?

The notion that social life in general, and family life in particular, is normatively regulated is not new or especially illuminating by itself. Sociologists such as Merton (1949) have commonly been more interested in determining why a person or group would violate institutional norms and behave in a deviant fashion than in addressing the question of why one set of social norms exists rather than some other. Of course, the functionalists answered this question with their list of functional prerequisites, which largely begged the question of why one particular set of norms has become institutionalized rather than some other set. The partial answer proposed below is that other social institutions must coordinate their norms with those of the family in order to have some degree of organized behavior in the social system. This is an incomplete answer to the question. A complete answer demands a view of social ecology that does not yet exist and is certainly beyond the scope of the present work.

A "social institution" is the set of norms regulating one relatively well-delineated area of social life. In regard to family life, the social institution of the family contains the norms regulating and defining mating, descent, socialization, and nurturance—in short, the norms governing affinal and consanguineal relationships over time. The fact that all the areas of family life are regulated over time simply takes into consideration that individuals age (mature), and that the social groups they form do the same. Thus, an important aspect of institutional norms is that they are age- and stage-graded in respect to both individuals and groups. This point is equally valid for other social institutions, such as politics and education.

There are subsets of norms within the institution of the family that govern three levels: individuals within the family, family subunits (dyads, triads, etc.), and the family as a unit. For example, a norm regarding mate selection is largely aimed at the individual, with the group supplying the sanctions. The norms constructing the role relationship of husband and wife govern household division of labor and are sanctioned by both the kin and larger society. The norms regulating family size and reproduction govern the number and timing of children. Sanctions for a family result from its coordination with other social-institutional norms. Note that all of these units (i.e., individual, subset, and family) age and mature, and hence must be governed by age- and stage-specific norms.

Aldous (1978) points out that these age-graded norms for family relationships must coordinate with one another; otherwise, too much role conflict and stress would result. Aldous (1978, pp. 128–130) shows graphically how the subcareers of marriage relations, sibling relations, and parental relations are age-graded and synchronized with one another so that a pile-up of stress is avoided. Hogan (1978) does much the same thing, except that his arguments pertain to the correspondence necessary between the norms of various social institutions.

Hogan (1978) argues that each individual passes through many age-graded and stage-graded social institutions during a lifetime. These age-graded norms are essential to the functioning of the sector of social life regulated by each institution, since the norms allow for the progressive development of knowledge, skills, and expertise. These norms must be organized between the various institutions as well as within them. Not only are expectations in a social institution usually tied to the appropriate maturation level for the individual or family; the sum total of expectations across institutions is linked to the expected capacity of the individual or family. For example, the probability that a family will simultaneously experience the death of the husband, the birth of the first child, the parents' last year of high school, a parent's beginning a job as an executive, a move to a new house, and the deaths of grandparents is low, partially because many of these events are regulated by age-graded norms of institutions that are coordinated with the norms of other institutions.

One particular set of norms that has been of some interest to developmental researchers is that of the institutional norms regulating the sequencing of events. Hogan (1978) suggests that when an individual gets out of "synchrony" with the normative sequence in one institutional career, the sequencing of events (career) in other institutional sectors will be thrown out of synchrony as well. One long-term consequence of such dysynchrony is that there are disruptions in careers. Thus, in some regards, these later-life career disruptions can be conceptualized as a type of aggregate or institutional sanction. For example, if a male does not sequence his work and education so that work follows completion of education, he is more likely to experience disruptions in his marital life (Hogan, 1978). Institutional norms and social organizations are geared to, for example, adolescents' being in high school, mothers' being relatively young, and men's being the principal wage earners. It is not surprising that when expectations are moved from one age to another, others (such as spouses) have their age and stage expectations disappointed.

The idea that there are both intra- and interinstitutional norms governing the sequencing of events in the life course has been challenged by Marini (1984). She bases her criticism on the lack of evidence for positive or negative sanctions for sequencing patterns. Furthermore, Marini argues that variations in sequencing by social class and ethnicity tend to cast doubt on the existence of one dominant pattern of sequencing as being the "norm." She cites the work of Modell (1980) to show that behavior changes often precede normative change, so that using sequencing behavior to indicate norms may not be valid.

Although Hogan and Astone (1986) have responded briefly to Marini's criticisms, a more detailed discussion is needed for these rather serious criticisms of the institutional-norms approach to sequencing. In large part, Marini's criticism is inappropriate for the level of analysis. Her criticisms are founded upon an indicator of social norms that is appropriate at the group level, but not at the aggregate or the institutional level of analysis. A "norm" may be indicated by the approval–disapproval evaluation of a group and associated sanctions (Gibbs, 1965; Marini, 1984); in this case, group sanctions indicate the norms. This is appropriate at the group level of analysis. However, the indication of norms at the aggregate level is the modal pattern of behavior. To the degree that there is variation from this modal pattern, there is an indication of the strength or weakness of the norm. Both of these ways of indicating a social norm are valid at the appropriate level of analysis. Both are indicators of a common construct of social norms as rules for behavior. To return to the analogy of the chess game introduced in Chapter 3, we might identify the rules of the game by when the players call each other "cheaters" instead of continuing to play; this would be the group-level indicator of the rules (norms). However, one could observe the moves and infer the rules of the game over a large number of games; this would be the aggregate-level indicator of the norms. Marini mistakenly views one of these indicators as valid and the other as invalid because she fails to identify the levels of analysis at which each is appropriate. Moreover, the sanctions at the aggregate level are revealed as more universal and general than those at the group level. Sanctions at the aggregate level are revealed as differential structural benefits and different life chances.

The idea that there are sanctions, both positive and negative, for conforming or not conforming to one institutional pattern of event sequencing (career) implies that the family career is normatively regulated. However, the family career must contain some flexibility in order to weather the random shocks that may occur, as, for example, during wars and depressions. Furthermore, there must be some capacity for institutional changes in norms. The notions of shocks to the system and capacity to incorporate adaptation suggest several hypotheses. The capacity of the institution of the family to adapt to changes in other social institutions, and in the social system in general, is most likely to be increased through a change in the norms regulating the family. These norms change through positive sanctions accruing to certain deviant family careers. One such deviant career is that originally followed by professionals who, because of their long tutelage, delayed marriage and childbirth. This deviant career had the positive consequences of higher earnings, smaller families, and greater social mobility. Over a few decades, this career, though still deviant from the majority, is increasing in popularity and may indicate a change in the norms governing the sequencing and timing of family events.

The example above raises one last issue in regard to institutional norms governing family life. There are norms that regulate which *events* are required, permitted, or forbidden. Likewise, there are norms that regulate the *order* of events or the sequencing of events for the family. And, lastly, there are norms regulating the *timing* of events. The timing of events, however, can mean either the age at which one should experience the event or the duration of time between events. These two meanings of the timing of events are conceptually separable, but empirically they are difficult to separate because of the underlying dimension of time. Conceptually, if a process is developmental, then the duration of time spent in a stage should indicate the time spent in the developing process. It is doubtful that this is such a neat monotonic relation, since many developmental processes (e.g., the learning curve) are nonmonotonic and curvilinear. Clearly, we cannot say that the longer a child spends in first grade, the more ready that child is for second grade. Nor can we say that the longer two people are married, the more ready they are for children. However, it is possible to assert that with both stage- and age-graded norms and event-related norms, the probability of a state transition is dependent on the duration of time in the present state. This may at times indicate that a relatively short duration of time in a state is associated with a high probability of transition, whereas a long duration of time in a state may be associated with a lower probability of transition. Such would seem to be the case with family formation—moving from marriage to the birth of a child.

CONCLUSION

The fit between the theoretical assumptions and propositions set forth in this chapter and the semi-Markov model appears to be a relatively good one. However, there is always the chance of mis-specification of the model. There are hazards in this regard from several sources. The theory is not as precise and well formed as it could be. For example, there is some considerable vagueness in the fifth proposition which is that previous stages influence present stages. Whether this "influence" is at most a dependence on the previous state or is some other type of dependence is unspecified. The model supposes that this assumption corresponds to the Markov assumption; however, this may not be the case. Another source for possible errors in specification may be the choice of the model. Although the theory clearly indicates a stochastic process, there are several other stochastic models that might be appropriate. For example, a model that depends on the current state alone, rather than on the duration in the current state, might be a contender.

The arguments for the fit between model and theory appear to be strong ones. These arguments serve to clarify what may be meant by vague statements in the theory. The assumptions and propositions taken together form an overall picture of the process of family development that is reflected by the model. At the same time, the model suggests new dimensions perhaps not previously considered by the theory. For instance, some common derivations from a Markov process are the mean time spent in a state, the risk or hazard of leaving a certain state, and the equilibrium distribution of the process. These mathematical patterns may suggest further substantive theoretical propositions.

It must be admitted that the substantive theory of family development is not fully represented by the nine assumptions and propositions identified in this chapter. Other authors, such as Rodgers (1973), have focused on the role relationships and the internal structure of the family over time. There are a large number of possible assumptions and propositions in regard to the internal structure and roles in the family. The choice not to include these points is based on three considerations. First, the theory views the principal unit of analysis as the family, and not subunits such as role relationships. Second, there already exist excellent discussions in this regard. Other authors (Rodgers, 1973; Aldous, 1978) have discussed these role relationships in considerable depth and detail.

The third consideration is this: It seems, as previously asserted in Chapter 3, that the more general levels of analysis constrain the more specific levels, but that the reverse is seldom the case. Thus, the aggregate level reflects the norms of the social institution of the family. The internal-subunit level is bounded by (1) the family as a whole unit; (2) the aggregate behavior of families in terms of conformity and deviance; and (3) the norms of the social institutions. For example, a young newly married couple may decide to wait a couple of years for the relationship to "cement" before they have children. The spouses may feel that they are making a unique decision based on their particular circumstances and interaction. However, an examination of the social norms using aggregate data reveals that their "decision" in fact conforms to aggregate behaviors based on the institutional timing norms. These institutional norms may be expressed by the general social system via socialization, or may be expressed by the closer context of kin. The spouses' perception that their decision is their own, though not mistaken, is thus sociologically unimportant in comparison to the normative structure. Therefore, the assumptions and propositions representing the substantive theory of family development in this chapter are the most general and useful for the more detailed analyses to follow.

CHAPTER 5

Methodological Issues: Models and Data

In the preceding chapter, the relationship between the substantive theory and the model has been examined. This chapter considers the relationship between the model and data. Thus far, a substantive theoretical interpretation has been linked to a specific mathematical model. This theoretically interpreted model serves to illuminate the substantive theory, as well as to suggest possible consequences that might not be so readily apparent in the substantive theory. The present chapter examines the relation between the model and data. This relation is a complex one, composed of the model's constraints on data collection and research design and the statistical analysis of data once collected.

The first part of the relation between model and data is the way in which it constrains the acquisition of data. For example, the semi-Markov model introduced in the preceding chapter carries with it assumptions about the form of data. The model supposes that we are dealing with a finite set of mutually exclusive and exhaustive states. The transitions between these states must be countable as either events or changes in state. Therefore, an individual or family can be counted as being in a state or not in a state at any particular time. These assumptions suggest that the data should be frequency data over time. It also seems evident that the data must be composed of successive observations on the same unit of analysis (a family or individual) over time. Thus, it seems that data for this model should be collected longitudinally.

A second aspect of the relation between model and data is the testing of core assumptions of the model. The most significant assumption of the semi-Markov model is that the probability of moving to another state is dependent on the time spent in the current state. This is a more specific version of the general Markovian assumption that the probability of moving to a new state is contingent only on the current state. The specific version of this assumption nicely formalizes the substantive theoretical definition of development. Clearly, if this assumption does not hold for longitudinal data on family state transitions, then both the appropriateness of the model and the adequacy of the theory are thrown into question. Hence, another factor in the relation between model and data is the testing of key assumptions.

The part of the relationship between a model and data that is perhaps most familiar to readers is the use of the model as a predictive device. This entails using the data to estimate the parameters of the model and then testing the estimated model as to its probable "fit" with data. The major problems in this area involve the ways in which unbiased estimates can be computed. The testing of the model is dependent on the estimation of empirical parameters from the data. However, some key assumptions, such as the Markovian assumption, can be tested without recourse to the estimation of all the parameters of the model. In fact, often a more specific case of the model is used rather than the general semi-Markov model. As previously mentioned, the semi-Markov model represents a family of models that includes such models as the Poisson and discrete-time Markov models. One or more of the models from this family may often be easier to use than the more general semi-Markov model. The more general semi-Markov model has, however, the distinct advantage that it is theoretically interpretable.

The purpose of this chapter is not to review the current state of developmental methodologies. Several excellent texts are available that devote the requisite space to such a complex subject (e.g., Miller, 1987). The purpose of this chapter is to discuss those issues that arise in the application and testing of the particular formulation of the theory of family development that has been advanced here. Some of these issues, such as problems with model identification and estimation, have already been alluded to briefly here. One issue that becomes important in regard to constraints on data collection and design is the acquisition of data as "states" or as "events." The observation of events for a unit of analysis (either the individual or the family) has distinct advantages over the observation of states. This chapter examines these issues, as well as the data collection and design constraints.

MODELS

Coleman (1981), after introducing the general semi-Markov model, suggests that "This model as it stands, for all but the richest forms of data, remains too general for use" (p. 10). Coleman's strategy is to utilize restricted versions of the general model that do not demand such rich data. The general model demands data indicating the duration of each individual's occupancy of each state and the exact times of transitions. Sometimes these detailed data are available for analysis, as in the case of life event histories. But often our observations lack at least some aspects demanded by the model.

As noted above, several more restricted models are part of the "family" of models identified with the general semi-Markov model. Some of these are renewal processes, proportional-hazards models, and discrete-time Markov models. Moreover, many of these models have both discrete- and continuous-time versions. A complete review of all of these models is beyond the scope of this study. More detailed discussions are to be found in Coleman (1981), Tuma and Hannan (1984), and Allison (1984). However, the discussion that follows may be enriched by some examples of these more restricted models and how they operate.

The most simple restricted model is the two-state model discussed by Coleman (1981). Imagine a continuous-time process where the transition rate between two states is constant or stable (stationary) over time for all individuals (i.e., it is homogeneous). For example, the two states can be "married" and "not married." Note that, like all defined states, these are exclusive and exhaustive. It is clear from these states that an individual can get married, divorced, and remarried, thus completing two transitions (i.e., the transition from "married" to "not married" and from "not married" to "married"). The simple model can be expressed as follows:

$$dp/dt = -qp \tag{1}$$

where p = the probability of being married
$1 - p$ = the probability of being not married
q = the transition rate from married to not married

It can also be expressed as a continuous-time process:

$$q = \lim_{\Delta t \to 0} \frac{r(\Delta t)}{\Delta t} \tag{2}$$

(Coleman, 1981, p. 11)

This model contains the discrete-time Markov process, represented in matrix notation as follows:

$$p(t) = p(0)\ r(t) \qquad (3)$$

where $p(t)$ = is the probability of being married at time 1
$p(0)$ = the probability of being married at time 0
$r(t)$ = where the log $r(t) = qt$

(Coleman, 1981, p. 14)

Both of these formulas indicate that the key ingredient to the model is the transition rate between states or the instantaneous transition rate for continuous-time processes. Coleman (1981) and Allison (1984) suggest that the transition rate be decomposed into a linear-effects model similar to regression models. The general form of this model is as follows:

$$\log r_{ij}(t) = a_{ij}(t - t') + b_{ij}x \qquad (4)$$

where $\log r = a(t - t') + bx$
x is a set of explanatory variables
t' is the time of the last transition, and
$a\ (t - t')$ is an unspecified function often treated as a constant constrained

(Allison, 1984, p. 58)

This type of model allows the transition rate to be treated as determined by various attribute variables such as occupation and age, as is often done in sociological inquiry. The difference here is that what is being explained is the rate of change from one state to another. In our example, what would be explained are two rates: the rate of change from "married" to "not married" and the rate of change from "not married" to "married."

Rather than enter a discussion at this point on which models serve what purposes and how they constrain data collection, I now turn to a topic that has been briefly discussed in Chapter 4: the relation between states and events. The reason for turning to this topic at this point is that these two different approaches, though complementary, necessitate somewhat different models and modes of inquiry.

STATES AND EVENTS

In Chapters 3 and 4, the distinction has been made between "stage" ("state") and "event." A stage or state is a qualitatively distinct period in the life of an individual or family. An event is a particular point in time marking the transition between stages or states. Accordingly, events separate and demarcate stages. Stages represent relatively uniform tasks and demands on the individual or family. An example of this distinction is the event of the birth of the first child to a couple. This event separates and delimits the two adjacent stages of "childless couple" and "couple with a new child." The roles and tasks for the childless couple are concerned with the marital relationship and the household. With the addition of a child, the couple becomes a dyad within the three-person family group; there are new tasks, such as the care and nurturance of an infant; and the new social roles of father and mother are added to the roles of husband and wife.

Clearly, the concepts of event and stage (state) are complementary. However, the semi-Markov model discussed thus far emphasizes the state or stage. There are several theoretical and practical problems with the state or stage approach. First, there is the theoretical problem previously mentioned in Chapter 4—namely, that there is no commonly agreed-upon set of states or stages that represents family development. Of the many different stage conceptions cited by Aldous (1978), none has received universal endorsement from family scholars. Even more important is the fact that none of the existing schemata are exhaustive of the empirical diversity of family forms. That is, these existing schemata fail to include stages that are relevant to single-parent families or to remarried or blended families (Borne et al., 1979; Ahrons & Rodgers, 1987, p. 22). The existing stage schemata, with the exception of the most simplistic, are not mutually exclusive. As previously discussed, a family may occupy two or more states at the same point in time. For example, the stages of "families with preschool children" and "families with school-age children" clearly are not mutually exclusive, since a family often contains both preschool and school-age children. Only the most simplistic and trivial of stage conceptions, such as "expansion," "stability," and "shrinkage," are not subject to these problems. Theoretically, neither the internal microtheoretical versions of family development such as that developed by Rodgers (1973) nor the macrotheoretical approaches such as that of Glick (1977) have solved this problem. In fact, authors representing the macrotheoretical perspective often rely on the event approach instead of the stage approach.

In addition to the theoretical problems with the stages concept, there are some important practical advantages of using observations on events rather than on stages. Coleman (1981) points out that the observation of events provides richer information than does the observation of states. The observation of a stage or state can only tell us whether a family or individual is in the state. By contrast, observation of events tells us exactly the point of transition between two states, thus yielding information about the previous state, the current state, and the exact time of the transition. Coleman suggests that this greater yield of information is a distinct advantage to the observation of events over stages.

A second practical consideration is that it is easier to collect data on events than on stages or states. For example, available public records often contain dates of status changes, such as the date of marriage and birth of the first child. These events are more readily available to researchers than are stages or states. Furthermore, the dates and numbers of events are often more easily incorporated into survey instruments than are questions regarding the "qualitatively distinct stages" of family life.

The general stochastic process model contains more restricted models that are appropriate for event analysis. For example, the Poisson process can be applied to the occurrence of an event; hazards models are also appropriate for the analysis of event data. Thus, the general model has the scope to deal with the observation of events as well as the observation of states. In addition, it is possible in many cases to use a variant of regression analysis for event data (e.g., Allison, 1984). Clearly, the theoretical and practical advantages to the observation of events rather than of stages or states are compelling.

PARAMETER ESTIMATION

Regardless of whether observations are made of events or of stages, some general considerations regarding the estimation of the parameters of models should be addressed at this point. The empirical estimation of parameters is a basic step in the testing of any model's "fit" with data. Theoretical guidelines are seldom available as to the parameters, so, in general, the strategy used is to estimate them from existing empirical data. This means that the estimates and test of the model are contingent on the validity and accuracy of the data, *and* on the type of estimation procedure. This second contingency is perhaps not as equivocal as it might appear, since estimates derived by different approaches often do not differ greatly.

There are three major approaches to the estimation of parameters for the class of models discussed here: estimation by moments, maximum likelihood, and partial likelihood. (Note that least squares, the fourth common type of estimation approach, is not appropriate for nonlinear models.) The method of maximum likelihood is by far the most often used. It involves choosing as estimates those values that maximize the probability of the observed data from which the estimates are being computed. Partial-likelihood estimation, originally developed by Cox (1975), represents a useful alternative, especially when data are missing or censored. The computation of such values is involved, and a full discussion of it is beyond the scope of this work; luckily, however, this form of estimation is now available in several computer packages. Interested readers should see Coleman (1981) and Tuma and Hannan (1984) for more detailed discussions.

One of the major stumbling blocks to the estimation of event data has been the fact that almost always the observations are "censored." This is the case when the data are truncated either at the beginning of the process ("left-censored") or at the time of the study or last panel ("right-censored"). The censoring problem is endemic to research on family development and to research testing dynamic models. For example, imagine that we want to study family formation, so we draw a sample of newlyweds and follow them for 5 years. At the end of the study, 5 years later, some of the newlyweds have had three children, some have had two children, some have had one child, and some have had none. We do not know, for instance, whether the couples having no children will have children or not. Nor do we know whether those with three children will continue their fertility. The conclusion of the study has truncated or censored the last state, in that we do not know how long it will last. This is an example of right-censored data. On the other hand, left-censored data would be obtained if we were to begin a study with a random sample of families. Even in the unlikely case that all these families were in the same initial stage, they would be at different points in that state or stage, and the length of time in the state would be truncated.

Tuma and Hannan (1984) suggest that there are three possible approaches to the censoring problem. First, we can ignore the censored states at both the beginning and end of our data and analyze only those states that are complete. Second, we can make the assumption that states begin and end when the observation period starts and ends. Third, we can adopt an estimation procedure that adjusts to the censoring by assuming that the same stochastic process applies across all states. All three of these approaches to censored data have been used by researchers; however, Tuma and Hannan argue that the third alternative is the most advantageous, since it avoids data loss and yields unbiased estimates for parameters when relatively large samples are used. They have developed maximum-likelihood procedures for both right- and left-censored data. The interested reader should see Tuma and Hannan (1984, pp. 116–154) for a detailed discussion of these procedures.

The problem of censored data applies to a lesser degree to event data. This is so because for formal purposes events can be considered as instantaneous points, unlike stages or states, which are occupied over a period of time. This does not mean that event analysis is without its problems; rather, the problems of estimation are different. Cox (1972, 1975) has addressed the problem of estimating parameters for models where data include the sequence of events but not the exact times of events. His partial-likelihood approach deals with this particular problem, which is often encountered in event analysis. The reader is referred to Coleman (1981, pp. 177–225) for both a discussion of this technique and a computer program for estimation of such parameters.

METHODS FOR EVENT DATA

The foregoing discussion has raised a number of issues, such as the censoring of data, that serve to guide researchers in the design of studies into family development. It has also raised several choices for the researcher, including units of analysis and units of observation. This section explores some of these options and the attendant design considerations.

The first consideration facing the researcher is the choice of the unit of analysis. As outlined in Chapter 3, there are several possible levels of analysis:

The individual
The dyad or triad (or other family subunit)
A family
Families (aggregate)
The institution of the family (i.e., norms)

Not all of these five levels of analysis are also the units on which observations or measurements can be made. A *level* of analysis is different from the *unit* of observation. The level represents the class or set of such units, and hence is a more abstract notion than the unit of analysis or observation. For example, the individual level of analysis represents the set of individual human beings as well as individual dogs, individual cells as well as individual chromosomes. Within the research focus of the family, a particular unit of observation at the individual level of analysis would be an individual member of a family. Individual units of observation can, in the aggregate, represent the institutional or aggregate level of analysis. The institutional level of analysis is composed of observations on individuals, on subunits of the family, and the aggregate of families from which norms can be inferred. The observation or measurement is made on the aggregate pattern, such as the modal event sequence. This aggregate pattern represents the unit of observation for the institutional level and the analysis of norms at this level. Hence, for the study of the family, there are really five units of measurement and observation related to each level of analysis: the individual, the family subunit, a family group, aggregations of these units, and the patterns of aggregations.

Each of these units can be investigated over time. However, not all of the dimensions of each unit of analysis represent elements of family development. For instance, many dimensions of the individual unit of analysis, such as income and occupation, must be considered as *exogenous* to the process of family development. That is, they must be viewed as coming from an institutional sector other than the family, even though they undoubtedly have an effect on family development.

When researchers of family development select the concept of "event" as the research domain, they have several choices as to variables within the event domain. There are several dimensions along which events may be measured, despite the fact that the concept is discrete and qualitative. These dimensions include the following:

1. The occurrence of the event
2. The frequency of the event
3. The sequence or order of events
4. The timing of the event
   a. The age of the unit of analysis at which the event occurred
   b. The chronological time of the event
   c. The duration of time between events

Each of these dimensions may be used without reference to the others. However, much more is to be gained by using multiple dimensions in any given analysis. Research into cohabitation serves as a good example. The event of interest is whether or not a couple has cohabited. Obviously, the length of cohabitation is an important variable, as is the next adjacent event (e.g., marriage or another cohabitation). Only when several dimensions are used in the analysis can important questions be answered, such as "Do people who cohabit have longer marriages than those without the experience of cohabitation?" The procession of events implies a procession of stages, which, in turn, implies roles and norms governing behavior. In order to examine this procession, several of these dimensions must be used for any given analysis. One of the most widely used approaches has been the study of event sequences.

EVENT SEQUENCES AND THE FAMILY CAREER

An "event sequence" is composed of the chronologically ordered events that have occurred for an individual or family over a specific period of time. As suggested above, the time period may be specified in several ways. The time period can be specified as a historical period, such as World War II or 1920–1930. The time period may also be specified by the age of the unit of analysis. For example, we could examine all the events occurring in families between 3 and 10 years from the date of their inception. Still another way in which the time period may be specified is by the time of study (or "panels") in longitudinal data collection (e.g., Teachman, 1982).

The analysis of event sequences has important theoretical implications. The concept of the family career is central to the theory of family development. Theoretically, the family career is the sequence of stages over time that an individual experiences, that a family traverses, or that families tend to follow. At the institutional level of analysis, the sequence of events that families (in the aggregate) tend to follow represents the path or sequence that is normatively defined as the way in which family life "should" proceed. The family career may be normatively defined as a particular order of events (or stages), the age at which a family or individual is to experience these events, and the length of time between events (or within each stage).

It is the normative order of events that has received the greatest attention from researchers. More specifically, researchers have been interested in the consequences of being out of step with the normative order of events. The theoretical ramifications of non-normative sequences of events are thought to be as follows: Once out of step with the normative order for the sequencing of events, the individual or family suffers the consequences of being out of step with all social institutions (e.g., family, education, and work) because of their stage- and age-graded organization of roles and norms. For instance, if an individual fails to sequence the completion of high school, first marriage, and first birth in the normative order, then subsequent family responsibilities may disrupt the completion of high school. If the person must return to an educational institution (which is not geared for older people, let alone mothers with children), this return may further put the individual out of step with the sequence of events in other institutions, such as work and family life. It would seem awkward to finish one's high school education while raising teenagers, or to attempt to maintain a full-time job while finishing school. The result might be time out of the labor force, which, in turn, could lead to yet other disruptions.

The non-normative sequencing of events is a form of deviance. It is at least a form of statistical deviance, in that it is not the way most people or families traverse their family life. In some cases it may be a conscious form of deviance, as when people choose to cohabit rather than to marry. And, in some cases, the deviance may be supported—in fact, encouraged—by other institutions. The delay of marriage and family life until a relatively old age by some professionals, so that they may complete their prolonged educational requirements, is one such example. Whether or not people in some such groups suffer from being out of step, even when it is encouraged by their profession, is a research question of some interest.

Two approaches are used in the analysis of deviant sequences. The more common approach is to treat various sequences as different levels of a categorical variable. Usually just a few events are specified as being the ones of interest. The various orders or permutations of these events are the levels of the variable. For example, Hogan (1978) was interested in the three events of first job, first marriage, and completion of education. The various orders of these three events served as the levels of the sequence variable (e.g., job, marriage, completion of education; or completion of education, marriage, job). Morgan and Rindfuss (1985) used a similar approach in their study of marital stability. The events they used were conception, marriage, and birth. This approach has been called the "Temporal Ordering Scale" by Hogan (1978). Although it bears little resemblance to a metric scale, the name is useful for distinguishing this approach from the second approach to the study of sequences of events.

The second approach is one I have developed (White, 1987a). This approach, unlike the Temporal Ordering Scale, has been devised to measure the *degree of deviance* from the dominant sequence pattern or career. This measurement approach is called the "Career Conformity Scale" and is a quasi-metric scale. The scale is constructed by beginning with the frequencies for all events regardless of order. Next, the frequencies for all sequences of events are computed. From these two sets of frequencies, events and sequences, the scale can be computed. First, the most frequently occurring sequence of events (modal sequence) is identified. Each position in the ordering is assigned its frequency as a score, and a total score is computed by adding all of the scores across all events.

To take the events that Morgan and Rindfuss (1985) used in their study as an example, the modal sequence would be the sequence of marriage followed by conception followed by birth. An instance of a deviant case would be conception followed by marriage followed by birth. In order to use the Career Conformity Scale, the frequencies of all events (marriage, conception, and birth) in the first position in the ordering would be examined. We already know that marriage is the most frequent event from the modal sequence, but we do not know how deviant other events are at this point in time. So it could be that premarital conceptions are very frequent compared to marriages or very infrequent. The comparison of the frequencies would indicate the degree of conformity to the modal pattern. The frequencies for all positions are then summed to represent the conformity–deviance for each individual (or family) over time. This score tells how deviant (low score) or conformist (high score) each person's career or sequence of events is. The usefulness of this approach is primarily in relation to Hogan's (1978) hypothesis that the more out of step one becomes, the greater are the negative consequences in relation to other institutions later in life. The Career Conformity Scale and this hypothesis are discussed in much greater detail in Chapter 10.

Both approaches to the measurement of sequences of events have strengths and weaknesses. The Career Conformity Scale has the advantage that data move from frequencies to a quasi-metric; thus, analysts may use statistical tools such as linear regression. On the other hand, log-linear models can be used with Hogan's Temporal Ordering Scale if the number of categories is small relative to sample size. This constraint is brought about not only because of a loss of degrees of freedom, but by the much more significant limitation of not having empty cells. This is such a problem that, even with large samples containing a few categorical independent variables, analysis may become impossible.

A distinct advantage of the Temporal Ordering Scale over the Career Conformity Scale is that it retains the exact events in each sequence. This is an advantage in that inspection may show one particular event to be common to several different orderings or sequences. The Temporal Ordering Scale maintains a close contact with the original events, whereas with the Career Conformity Scale all one has is a score with its distribution and moments. It becomes difficult to identify particular events that fall in particular temporal positions, which may be of special significance in relation to a dependent variable.

The strengths and weaknesses of each approach suggest that they should be used in conjunction in the analysis of sequence data. Certainly, there is no contradiction between the two approaches. Each approach reveals a different dimension of event sequencing. The Temporal Ordering Scale reveals the exact events and their order. The Career Conformity Scale deals with the notion of the normative character of these sequences, and measures the statistical deviation from the statistical norm as a way of operationalizing this concept. Thus, both approaches yield important information for the researcher of families' developmental sequences or careers.

DURATION, AGE, PERIOD, AND COHORT

A key assumption of both the model and the theory is that family change is developmental only if the probability of that change depends on the duration of time spent in the preceding stage. How does this assumption translate into the analysis of events? Since events formally represent instantaneous points of transition between stages, then a sequence of adjacent events represents $n + 1$ stages. The duration of time between adjacent pairs is the duration in the state, even if the stage or state cannot be theoretically identified. Thus, event analysis offers a means to test the assumptions regarding the process of family development, while temporarily skirting the thorny theoretical issue of developing a set of exhaustive and exclusive theoretical stages. But, since events are defined as points between stages, such a strategy can only be temporary at best.

There are several problems with assuming that a process is duration-dependent. The major problem in this respect is that since duration is a time measure, a number of other processes and effects could account for what might be perceived as duration dependence. Most developmental researchers are familiar with three of these time-associated variables: age, cohort, and historical period (e.g., Baltes, 1968; Baltes & Schaie, 1973). In addition to these three, some scholars would add the variable of "experience" (Tuma & Hannan, 1984). There has been much discussion of problems surrounding the separation of these effects, and it is important to examine these issues briefly in regard to the theoretical assumption of duration dependence as the defining criterion for a developmental process.

The assumption of duration dependence, as stated earlier, is the assumption that the probability of moving to a state is dependent on the length of time spent in the current state. Some theorists have assumed that a family must reach a level of functioning or adaptation to the normative demands for each stage before a transition to the next stage is normatively permitted or required. This idea was originally attached to the notion of "developmental tasks" associated with each stage. However, the inability of family scholars to specify the stages of family development, let alone the developmental tasks within each stage, makes the notion of developmental tasks descriptive at best. It is descriptive of the process of family members' learning and coordinating new family roles (either because of changes in role content as a result of age-grading or because of new roles, as with the arrival of the first child), and establishing competence in the performance of those roles. This means that duration dependence pertains in the aggregate to the phenomena associated with the social-psychological process of group learning and adaptation to family roles and norms.

There are, of course, other types of learning and adaptation to social roles going on for individuals, which may be confounded with the learning of family roles. For example, there seems little doubt that extensive work experience in the administration of an office may assist one in adapting to the demands of administering a home, and may thus speed up the process for this individual, if not for the family as a group. This confounding effect is that of experience. "Experience" can also mean an individual's exposure to various states prior to a given state (Tuma & Hannan, 1984). In this sense, a family or individual may have traversed many family states prior to the current state, and the cumulative effect is that of experience. Duration dependence is often confounded with experience of previous states, since as one gains experience in adapting to demands, the learning or experience that takes place assists in adapting to the next set of demands. There seems no single methodological approach that can completely remove this threat. One strategy that can be employed is to examine the sequences of events over a family or individual history, to ascertain whether the present state is more dependent on different sequences than on the immediately preceding state. Nevertheless, this technique will only partially address the problem of confounding experience with duration dependence. Other partial solutions depend on the research interest. Again, however, there is no single complete way to eliminate experience as a competing explanation for our theoretical interpretation of duration dependence.

Age is a variable that is easily confounded with duration, since both have time as an underlying dimension. One does not age without a change in time, nor does duration in a state vary except as time varies. Thus, this is a classic example of multicollinearity: The age of the family or individual and the duration of time in a state will always be correlated. As Tuma and Hannan (1984) point out, age is a variable that often stands for the effect of age-graded norms on behavior or the effect of situational changes such as institutional structures. For instance, age is a good predictor of employment, since the very young and very old are not employed. When the variables for which age serves as a proxy can be specified, then the confounding with duration is reduced. However, age also stands for maturation, a combination of physiological development and exposure or experience. In this second sense, age will, like experience, be confounded with duration of time in a state. One possible way of dealing with this problem is to sample different age groups over time as they move through the same set of states. This design strategy is discussed later in this chapter. It cannot remove the confound between age and duration completely, however.

The historical period in which an event has occurred may have an effect on the duration in a state. An example is the length of time young men were single during World Wars I and II. The historical period had a clear effect on the duration in that state. Historical period also captures some of the changes in institutional norms over time. The norms governing family life, for example, were different during the war periods. Thus, we find that period, age, and duration are confounded.

Birth cohort is correlated with both age and period. These cohort effects are usually thought to identify the normative culture in which a "generation" was raised. Computationally, it is easy to see that the present date minus birth year equals present age. Here, period, age, and cohort are linearly related. It is impossible to isolate the effect of any one of these from the effects of the others. Although some developmental scholars have thought that these effects could be separated by careful designs, it is now clear that this does not offer a true solution to the problem (e.g., Glenn, 1977; Tuma & Hannan, 1984).

Duration in a state shares most of these problems with age, period, and cohort. To some limited extent, it is possible to get an idea of how each of these functions, but never independently of the others. In fact, much of what we see appears to consist of interactions between these variables. A person's age determines what experiences are allowed by various social institutions at various periods in time; these experiences are related to the maturation and development of the individual; and all of these are related to the individual's duration in a given state. It is only by means of carefully designed studies that even an unclear indication of effects may be afforded.

RESEARCH DESIGN

There is a wealth of information on the subject of research designs for developmental research. This information, however, is distributed across several different academic areas, such as social gerontology, developmental psychology, and child development. The discussion to follow can be only a brief and selective introduction to some of the issues in regard to research designs for the study of family development. Interested readers should see Miller (1987) for a recent and more complete review of many of these issues.

Two basic research designs are used in the study of family development: longitudinal designs and cross-sectional designs. Although most researchers are familiar with these two designs, it is important to reassess them in terms of their appropriateness for the theory and models for family development. Furthermore, it is important to reassess the strengths and weaknesses of these designs in terms of how each deals with the problems of the confounded variables of duration, age, cohort, and period.

A "cross-sectional" design is one in which different samples are studied at different times, or, in the most restricted case, one sample is studied at one point in time. One of the major characteristics of a cross-sectional design is that individuals in one sample do not systematically appear in any subsequent samples. Several advantages of this design are immediately apparent. The expense involved is often not as great as in longitudinal and other designs. Also, this design avoids the problems of sample attrition that so often are found with longitudinal designs.

However, cross-sectional designs have a glaring weakness in research on family development. This weakness is that the theory and model specify a *process,* and a cross-sectional design cannot be used to examine the hypothesized process. For example, since we are interested in a family's duration of time in a stage, we might draw a sample of families in 1987 and a sample of families in 1988 and attempt to see how many families are still in a certain stage. However, no matter how well the two samples are matched, since they are different families we can have little confidence that we are observing a developmental process. For some research questions within the theory of family development, cross-sectional designs are appropriate. The question regarding correlates of a stage is one of these; research questions regarding exogenous variables associated with family events are also questions for which cross-sectional designs may be used.

In some types of research, use of cross-sectional designs may be necessary because doing a longitudinal design would simply take too much time. For instance, if one wanted to study the differences between new parents' anxiety with children and older, more experienced parents' anxiety, a cross-sectional approach might be used rather than a 10-year longitudinal study. However, a cross-sectional design would always confound the variables of age and cohort. That is, we would never be able to tell whether differences in anxiety between the sample of new and old parents were due to the difference in ages or to the fact that the groups also represent different cohorts raised with different attitudes and values toward child rearing. Needless to say, we also could not tell whether duration in the parental stage or age or cohort would be responsible for any differences that might exist. This confounding of these variables is endemic to the simple cross-sectional design.

The "longitudinal" design may, on the surface, seem to be the design strategy of choice for developmental researchers. Among theorists of family development, longitudinal research has often been seen as capable of answering the developmental questions that remain unanswered by cross-sectional approaches. Longitudinal research is the study of the same sample on at least two different occasions separated by a length of time. Although repeated-measures designs may seem to fit this definition, usually the period of time between tests is not deemed sufficiently long to qualify this research as longitudinal. The usual way in which longitudinal studies are conducted is to select a sample at a particular age or stage of development and then to test this sample at several time points, usually over a period of years. It is immediately obvious that this type of research is costly in both time and money, compared to cross-sectional research.

Many problems besides time and money plague longitudinal research. One of the best known of these problems is sample attrition. Over a long period of time subjects may become tired of the project, move to another location, die, or otherwise become lost to the sample. The sample thus becomes increasingly nonrandom, and conclusions become suspect. Another problem is that produced by repeated testing. For example, successive administering of a marriage satisfaction instrument not only may lead subjects to fill out the instrument in stereotypical ways, but may result in the subjects' being more aware of marital problems because of testing (reactivity).

Despite these problems, when we want to get information about a process, longitudinal designs are usually preferred (Wilson, 1975). This preference is based on the assumption that since a longitudinal design follows the same units of analysis over time, the changes observed in those units reflect the process. Thus, we expect that duration in a stage can best be measured longitudinally. However, there is a problem with when to take successive measures on what we assume to be a continuous process, since it is exceedingly likely that families or individuals will not shift stages at the same time. A more difficult problem is the confounding of the age of the unit of analysis and the historical period in which measures are taken. It may be impossible to tell whether changes in state are due to the maturation (age) of a family, to occurrences at the time of measurement (e.g., wars or depression), or to more subtle psychological influences (e.g., women's liberation or fear of AIDS). However, it is possible to separate age from duration in state, and thus to answer a question that is crucial to the theory of family development—that is, the semi-Markov assumption. One last problem with longitudinal research is that it seldom studies more than one age cohort over time, and thus the representativeness of its conclusions is limited to that specific age group. In the case of families, the same criticism would apply to a study where families are followed from a particular event such as a wedding day; the sample thus represents the cohort of families married in that specific year.

Several variants on the two basic designs, cross-sectional and longitudinal, address some of the specific problems plaguing the basic designs. The "time-lag" design is one in which a particular age group (e.g., 20-year-olds) is studied on successive occasions. So, for example, a time-lag design would study 20-year-olds in 1980, 1985, 1990, and 1995. Each sample would naturally be cross-sectional. As Miller (1987) points out, the time-lag design contains the confounding of cohort with the period at which the measurement was taken. On the other hand, the time-lag design helps address the confound between age and cohort (cross-sectional) and age and period of measurement (longitudinal). The time-lag design lacks one important characteristic for the testing of developmental propositions, and this is that it fails to get at the process within the unit of analysis.

Another variant of the basic cross-sectional design is the "cross-sectional/sequential" design. In this design, the usual cross-sectional sample is taken, but at several time points. Thus a researcher studying families might take a random sample of families in 1985 and again in 1990, using the same instruments and sampling procedures. Because at least two cohorts are sampled, this approach allows for at least some estimate of the cohort effect independent of the age effect—the typical confound of cross-sectional designs. However, as with its relatives, the time-lag design and traditional cross-sectional design, the cross-sectional/sequential design fails to study changes within a unit of analysis, and thus is less than successful for studying process.

A variant of the basic longitudinal design is the "longitudinal/sequential" design. This design, like all longitudinal designs, follows subjects over time. However, rather than just following one cohort over time, the longitudinal/sequential design follows at least two different cohorts at the same times. Thus, this design affords an opportunity to disentangle age and period, age and duration, and cohort and period. The distinct disadvantage of this design is its cost in time and money. In addition, the opportunity for sample attrition is magnified by having several age cohorts rather than one. Furthermore, the chance for variability as a result of normal attrition (e.g., attrition due to deaths) is more likely. As Glenn (1977) notes, this variability has yet to be dealt with statistically, and in fact there is some doubt as to whether it can be.

There is one last design to be discussed, but first a digression is necessary. Thus far in this discussion, we have seen that all the designs have problems. It must be admitted that perfect information cannot be obtained unless we can somehow deal with the variation resulting from mortality and mobility. This is unlikely. However, it is possible to gain some idea of what such information would look like. A common way to view developmental data is to represent it in a matrix, with the rows representing the birth cohorts and the columns representing the times of measurement (periods) (e.g., Glenn, 1977; Miller, 1987). The most complete data we could have would fill all the cells of such a matrix. All of the designs discussed here would only fill some of the cells by row (longitudinal) or by column (cross-sectional). Table 5.1 demonstrates such a matrix.

Inserted in the cells of this matrix are the ages of subjects or units of analysis. The age of a subject is, of course, computed by subtracting the birth date from the time of measurement. This matrix, following Miller (1987) and Glenn (1977), can be used to demonstrate each design discussed thus far. Any single row represents a simple longitudinal design over 30 years (1970–2000). Any single column represents a simple cross-section containing particular age groups. For instance, if a cross-sectional study were completed in 1970, it would contain ages from 10 to 40. The time-lag study can be represented as any diagonal line containing the same age group across times of measurement. The cross-sectional/sequential design can be represented by two or more columns. The longitudinal/sequential design can be represented by two or more rows. Clearly, the most complete data that could be had would fill all cells. But obtaining such data would be prohibited by both cost and time considerations.

The last design to be discussed is the "retrospective" design. A retrospective study is basically a one-point-in-time, cross-sectional survey in which the respondents are asked to recollect or recount events in the past. Because retrospective approaches yield information similar to that obtained in longitudinal studies, but unaccompanied by the costs

TABLE 5.1. Cohort and Period Matrix

	Time of measurement (period)			
Birth cohort	1970	1980	1990	2000
1930	40	50	60	70
1940	30	40	50	60
1950	20	30	40	50
1960	10	20	30	40

and time commitments of a longitudinal study, retrospective designs have become increasingly used by developmental researchers.

The type of information gathered by retrospective studies is *similar* but not *identical* to the type of information collected in longitudinal studies. The differences are worth noting. One important difference is that a longitudinal study actually takes measurements at different points in time, whereas the retrospective design relies on the self-report and recall of the respondents. Many scholars have noted that self-reports tend to be biased by social desirability (e.g., Ferber & Birnbaum, 1979). Even more criticism has been directed at the retrospective design's reliance on the respondents' recall. For example, Yarrow, Campbell, and Burton (1970) reported that present perceptions influenced recall of past events. Distortion of past events was most pronounced with attitudinal items. In general, it seems that respondents are more reliable in their recall of significant life events than of attitudes held at a previous time (Gutek, 1978). In fact, Finney (1981) suggests restricting questions in retrospective studies to simple, relatively objective matters, rather than complex issues or attitudes.

On the positive side, several compelling arguments favor retrospective designs for the study of family events. Since family events are supposed to be the transition points between stages of family life, they should be relatively significant to the respondents, and hence more accurately recalled than attitudes. In addition, Yarrow et al. (1970) suggest, checks on reliability may be added to insure the quality of the data. One such check is to ask the dates of events independently from the order of events. Clearly, the dates of events should indicate the order of events. It thus appears that at least some of the problems associated with recall can be addressed in retrospective studies of family events.

One of the major advantages of the retrospective approach is that it makes possible the acquisition of vast numbers of data on family and respondent history, which would otherwise be virtually impossible to acquire by means of longitudinal studies. Retrospective designs allow the researcher to complete most if not all of the cells in the matrix in Table 5.1. Given these advantages, it is little wonder that many cross-sectional studies now incorporate some retrospective questions and that several national census bureaus either have already implemented retrospective designs or are contemplating doing so (e.g., Canada, the United States, and the People's Republic of China).

The retrospective design does have drawbacks that make it inappropriate for some types of research (e.g., Cherlin & Horvich, 1980; Featherman, 1980). For instance, attitudinal researchers would be ill advised to use this approach. In addition, researchers using quantitative variables at either the interval or ratio level of measurement could no longer consider these as meaningful scales in a retrospective design (unless standardized across time, as economists do with 1970 pre-inflationary dollars). However, for the study of relatively important, objective events, the retrospective design seems to offer many of the advantages of the longitudinal design without the costs in time and money associated with longitudinal designs.

CONCLUSION

Several important topics have been covered in this chapter, and some summary of the conclusions reached in regard to the issues discussed is necessary. Briefly, the major points are as follows:

1. The semi-Markov model represents a family of models, some of which are appropriate for the analysis of events (e.g., Poisson) and some of which are appropriate for states (e.g., renewal).
2. The use in research of events rather than states is suggested for one major reason: A satisfactory theoretical specification of exclusive and exhaustive stages is not developed at this time and may not be developed for some time to come.
3. The problem of censored data will plague all longitudinal and retrospective research, but the problem varies in magnitude with the nature of the research question.
4. The notion of duration in a stage is definitionally tied to the meaning of development. However, only a partial empirical picture will be possible, because duration is necessarily related to other time-based variables (age, cohort, period, and experience).
5. Event sequences or orderings of events constitute one way to study the normative (institutional) nature of event sequences.
6. Although longitudinal/sequential designs are best for studying family process, retrospective designs may serve as good proxies when the research focus is on events rather than attitudes or psychological states.

These six conclusions from this chapter indicate that some important questions in the theory of family development can be addressed by the analysis of events using retrospective designs. This is not to say that all of the relevant research in this area should ideally be of this sort. Rather, this conclusion is based on the limitations placed on researchers by the present level of theory and the dual realities of time and funding.

The semi-Markov model does not appear to constrain research to the degree that theoretical and practical considerations do, mainly because the general model contains several more restricted but useful and applicable models. The works by Coleman (1981) and Allison (1984) are helpful in this regard. Hogan (1978, 1981) has laid the foundation for the analysis of orderings of events, and I have elaborated on this approach elsewhere (White, 1987a). It is now time to turn to empirical investigations to see what these can tell us in regard to family development.

PART III

EMPIRICAL EXPLORATIONS

CHAPTER 6

Family History Data

The purpose of this chapter is to introduce the two sets of data that are used in the subsequent chapters. The chapters to follow are concerned with testing and illustrating some critical aspects of the theory of family development; hence, the empirical data used for these tests are constrained by the assumptions discussed in the previous chapters. The most obvious constraint is that in order to study process rather than a particular point in time, either longitudinal or retrospective designs must be used. Both of the investigations that supplied the data sets used here employed retrospective designs. Apart from this similarity, there were many differences between these investigations, such as the data collection procedures, sampling methods, and target populations.

Both data sets consist of individuals' reports on family and work events. Since the individuals were reporting the events that *they* had experienced rather than those that their families had experienced, some caution is required in interpreting these reports as "family history" rather than as "individuals' history of family events." However, the reality is that an individual's history of family events is the best approximation available as an indication of a family's history. After all, if an individual experienced a "family event," then that event must have occurred for the family. Nonetheless, caution is necessary, especially in the specification of family events, so that such events are genuinely "family" and not "individual" events.

The two data sets, as noted, come from different sources. The Family History Survey was designed and the resulting data were collected by Statistics Canada in February 1984. With the assistance of Roy H. Rodgers, I designed the Family Structure and Family Career Project and collected the resulting data in June 1983. Both projects contain extensive family history data, as well as some point-in-time (cross-sectional) measures. A full discussion of each project, and some characterization of the data, are provided below.

THE FAMILY HISTORY SURVEY

Research Design and Procedure

The Family History Survey was initiated by Statistics Canada to assist in filling many of the gaps in our knowledge about families in Canada. Such gaps exist in part because the great bulk of research is cross-sectional and not longitudinal. However, the not insignificant costs associated with longitudinal designs act as a deterrent to such research. The strength of the retrospective design is that, while its costs are similar to those of other types of cross-sectional research, it provides data that are good substitutes for longitudinal data. Thus, Statistics Canada selected this approach for the acquisition of family data.

The population from which the sample was drawn was that of the Canadian Labour Force Survey.[1] The Labour Force Survey was a multi-stage area sample, stratified by economic region as well as by several other population units based on the census. Although the Labour Force Survey interviewed respondents 15 years of age and up, the Family History Project only sampled those respondents between 18 and 65 years of age. The very young (those aged 15–17) were excluded because they would not have had many family events as yet; in addition, there was the sensitive issue of asking very young people questions regarding births and common-law arrangements. Those respondents who were over 65 years of age at the time of the Labour Force Survey, 6 months prior to the Family History Survey, were also excluded from the sample. This was done because it was felt that for some respondents over 65 years of age, the recall of events and dates might be unduly taxing.

Another restriction on the Family History Survey was that certain groups were excluded from participation in the Labour Force Survey, and thus automatically would not appear in the Family History Survey. Those excluded were as follows: residents of both the Yukon and the Northwest Territories, armed forces personnel, all residents of Indian reserves, inmates of institutions, and foreign diplomats. Statistics Canada estimated that these excluded groups comprised approximately 2% of the population of Canada at that time.

The Labour Force Survey used a rotating sample; that is, one-sixth of the sample was rotated out of the sample each month and was replaced by a "fresh" group. The entire sample was thus different every 6 months. This rotation was aimed at the partial elimination of respondent fatigue and noncooperation. The Family History Survey used two different rotations for its sample: Males were from one rotation group and females from another. The sampling unit was the household. Therefore, it was possible that a female and a male from the same household could end up in the study. It is thus necessary to analyze the female and male samples independently.

The Family History Survey selected 16,000 potential respondents from the Labour Force Survey. This sample of potential respondents did not include those who refused to give the interviewers their telephone numbers at the outset or who did not have telephones. Burch (1985) estimated that these refusals comprised about 2% of the original sample. Telephone interviews were conducted by Statistics Canada interviewers other than those used in the Labour Force Survey, in order to assure respondents of confidentiality. There was a nonresponse rate of 12.7%, which resulted in a sample size of 14,004 individuals (approximately 6,750 males and 7,250 females).

The data were edited for consistency by Statistics Canada. For example, since dates for events were collected, it was possible to check the sequence of events as well as to check birth dates against one another. Where possible, standard imputation techniques were used to edit missing or suspect data. Inconsistent records were checked against the questionnaire.

Statistics Canada released the microdata tape and documentation for the Family History Survey in August 1985. The documentation cautions users that the sample weights should be used when one is concerned with generalizing to the population of Canada. These weights correct for urban-rural differences in representation, regional differences, and the variation in response rates. These weighted data are reported in this chapter. However, in subsequent chapters these sample weights are not used in the analyses where a particular nonrandom subsample is drawn in order to explore theoretical hypotheses or explorations. For instance, in order to examine the effect of different orders of events such as first marriage, first job, and first child, a subsample of all those who experienced all three events in any order must be formed. Because such a subsample is clearly not representative, no claim whatsoever is made in this regard, and the data analyzed are the actual individual responses rather than weighted data.

Description of the Sample

This section provides a general overview of the sample. In subsequent chapters, some subsample of this sample is generally used. For instance, only those cases in which certain events were experienced are examined in one of the later analyses. Since the overall sample supplies the cases for these subsamples, it is useful to provide some general idea of the characteristics of the entire sample. In order to do this, I now examine the weighted results of the survey, which are representative of the Canadian population.

The sample, as noted above, consisted of approximately 7,250 females and 6,750 males between the ages of 18 and 65. Table 6.1 shows that most of these people married at some point in their lives. Of the males and females between 50 and 64 years of age, over 93% had been married at some time in their lives. This percentage might be expected to be somewhat lower among people in the younger age groups, who may have been pursuing careers rather than marriage. However, even the percentage ever married in the group aged 30 to 39 was relatively high (85–88%). These data suggest that marriage is a significant life event for the great majority of Canadians.

The fact that many Canadians experience the event of marriage as did their parents does not mean that the institution is identical to the one in which they grew up. The fact that divorce had become more common and more accepted by the 1980s than it was in the 1960s is evidenced in Table 6.2. Clearly, the incidence of divorce had increased significantly

TABLE 6.1. Per Cent Ever Married by Number of Marriages, Age Group, and Sex, Canada, 1984

Sex and age group	Ever married	Number of marriages		
		One	Two	Three
Male				
18–29	33.9	33.2	0.7[a]	—[b]
30–39	85.0	79.7	5.3	—
40–49	92.0	84.3	6.9	0.8[a]
50–64	93.2	85.1	7.7	0.4[a]
All ages	70.7	65.9	4.6	0.2[a]
Female				
18–29	45.3	44.2	1.2	—
30–39	88.0	81.5	6.3	0.2[a]
40–49	93.4	84.9	8.1	0.3[a]
50–64	94.1	86.1	7.5	0.5[a]
All ages	75.8	70.5	5.1	0.2[a]

Note. From *Family History Survey* (Statistics Canada, Catalogue No. 99-955) by T. K. Burch, 1985, August, Ottawa: Statistics Canada. Copyright 1985 by the Minister of Supply and Services, Canada. Reprinted by permission.

[a]These percentages represent very few cases and therefore may contain a high level of error.

[b]The dash (—) in this and all other tables indicates no observation.

TABLE 6.2. Per Cent Ever Divorced by Age Group and Sex, Canada, 1984

	Male		Female	
Age group	Of total	Of ever married	Of total	Of ever married
18–29	1.4	4.1	3.7	8.2
30–39	9.9	11.7	13.8	15.7
40–49	12.8	13.9	15.0	16.1
50–64	8.1	8.6	9.1	9.7
All ages	7.1	10.1	9.4	12.4

Note. From *Family History Survey* (Statistics Canada, Catalogue No. 99-955) by T. K. Burch, 1985, August, Ottawa: Statistics Canada. Copyright 1985 by the Minister of Supply and Services, Canada. Reprinted by permission.

for those 49 years old and younger. The fact that the percentage divorcing between the ages of 18 and 29 was comparatively small is probably more an indication of the short time spent in marriage than of a decline in the divorce rate for this group. The number of years spent in marriage represents the length of time spent at risk of divorce. Although the relationship between risk and time married is probably not a simple monotonic function, it largely explains the lower incidence of divorce for this youngest cohort.

Yet another indication that the institution of marriage was different at the time of the survey than it was for earlier cohorts is the increased prevalence of cohabitation or common-law relationships prior to marriage. Table 6.3 shows that between 22% and 26% of those in the youngest age cohort were marrying partners with whom they had previously cohabited. The frequency of reported cohabitations for those in the oldest cohort was so small as to be unreported because of its statistical instability. Clearly, premarital cohabitation represents a change in the courtship pattern, and thus probably signifies changes in the institution of marriage. Most certainly, one of the changes may be the age at marriage if premarital cohabitation serves to delay marriage.

The average ages for cohabitation, marriage, and divorce were different for each age cohort. These differences are most probably due to two factors. One is that social norms change at points in time, and these point-in-time changes affect age cohorts at different ages. For example, as noted above, divorce became more socially acceptable and legally easier in the decade of the 1960s, and those in their 60s at the time of the survey were in their 40s then. Thus, this age cohort lacked at least 10 years' exposure to the same risk of divorce that younger cohorts would have had. The second factor is related to the more continuous nature of

TABLE 6.3. Per Cent Whose First Marriage Was to a Common-Law Partner, and Per Cent of Those Ever in a Common-Law Union Who Married a Common-Law Partner, by Age Group and Sex, Canada, 1984

Sex and age group	Of ever-married, percentage whose first marriage was to a common-law partner	Of those ever in a common-law union, percentage who married a common-law partner
Male		
18–29	26.6	46.1
30–39	10.2	52.4
40–49	2.1	41.5
50–64	. . .[a]	26.3
All ages	8.1	46.0
Female		
18–29	22.2	40.5
30–39	8.4	49.7
40–49	. . .[a]	43.3
50–64	. . .[a]	27.6
All ages	7.4	42.6

Note. From *Family History Survey* (Statistics Canada, Catalogue No. 99-955) by T. K. Burch, 1985, August, Ottawa: Statistics Canada. Copyright 1985 by the Minister of Supply and Services, Canada. Reprinted by permission.
[a]Due to a high standard error, these figures are not shown.

changes in social norms. Even though it is helpful in understanding "time-at-risk" phenomena to conceptualize normative shifts as occurring at a point in time, these normative shifts are often more gradual and continuous in nature. To continue with the example of divorce, more favorable attitudes toward divorce and divorced people evolved during the 1960s and the decades following. These norms changed gradually. Thus, the behavior of each age cohort was affected differentially, because those in the youngest cohort began their marriages with relatively liberal attitudes about divorce, whereas those in the oldest cohort began their marriages with distinctly less favorable norms. The effects of the norms with which one begins marriage, and the effects of changing norms during one's married years, both play a part in understanding divorce rates. The cohort differences seen here are thus due to a combination of the norms with which respondents began marriage and the different ages at which different cohorts experienced shifts in normative content. These differences are reflected in the different average ages at which the various age cohorts experienced different marital events (see Table 6.4).

The data from the Family History Survey also suggest that Canadian families are largely composed of natural children rather than

TABLE 6.4. Average Age at Various Marital and Family Events by Age Group and Sex, Canada, 1984

Sex and age group	First cohabitation	First marriage	First divorce	First widowed	Second marriage	Second divorce
Male						
18–29	21.2	22.1	24.5	—	26.5	—
30–39	25.9	23.6	29.5	29.7	30.3	31.8
40–49	33.4	24.6	35.5	36.7	36.3	39.9
50–64	44.7	26.2	42.9	46.8	43.1	48.2
All ages	26.4	24.4	34.4	45.2	36.7	41.0
Female						
18–29	20.5	20.8	24.5	22.3	25.0	—
30–39	25.6	21.9	29.3	28.9	29.5	33.9
40–49	32.9	21.9	36.1	34.8	35.5	38.7
50–64	39.9	23.3	41.5	46.8	41.3	50.5
All ages	24.7	22.1	33.3	43.5	34.9	42.4

Note. Average ages are shown only for the groups to which the events apply; that is, those who have ever married, ever divorced, ever remarried, and so on. Some respondents may belong to more than one group, and others to only one. That explains why some of the average ages do not fall in expected sequence. (For example, the average age at first divorce of females now aged 40–49 is 36.1 and at second marriage only 35.5.) From *Family History Survey* (Statistics Canada, Catalogue No. 99-955) by T. K. Burch, 1985, August, Ottawa: Statistics Canada. Copyright 1985 by the Minister of Supply and Services, Canada. Reprinted by permission.

adopted children or stepchildren. Table 6.5 shows that most of the Canadians surveyed had children of their own. Families with adopted children or stepchildren were infrequent; when such families were encountered, they tended to be small ones. The relatively small percentage of children reported for the youngest age cohort indicates that this group had probably not completed childbearing; it also may reflect the trend to reduce family size. At this time, it still remains to be seen whether or not these people will have substantially reduced fertility or simply delayed fertility compared to older cohorts.

These data suggest that courtship patterns are changing with the increased frequency of cohabitation, and that divorce continues to become more widely accepted and practiced. These changes in the development of families are accompanied by changes in the timing of when children leave the parental home. According to the survey, most children left the parental home by the age of 25, with only about 10% in the home after that age. Females left home earlier than males, probably because of their earlier age at marriage and earlier age at cohabitation. Stepchildren

TABLE 6.5. Per Cent Who Have Ever Raised Natural Children, Step-children, or Adopted Children by Age Group and Sex, Canada, 1984

Sex and age group	Natural children	Stepchildren	Adopted children[a]
Male			
18–29	22.0	1.4	. . .[b]
30–39	74.6	5.6	2.4
40–49	83.8	6.6	3.8
50–64	83.4	5.8	5.0
All ages	60.3	4.4	2.6
Female			
18–29	34.9	. . .[b]	. . .[b]
30–39	79.8	2.8	2.5
40–49	88.3	3.5	4.9
50–64	86.4	2.4	4.3
All ages	67.5	2.1	2.5

Note. From *Family History Survey* (Statistics Canada, Catalogue No. 99-955) by T. K. Burch, 1985, August, Ottawa: Statistics Canada. Copyright 1985 by the Minister of Supply and Services, Canada. Reprinted by permission.
[a]Not counting stepchildren who have been legally adopted.
[b]Due to a high standard error, these figures are not shown.

left the home earlier than did either natural or adopted children. For example, for the female parents with children between the ages of 15 and 19, only 57% of the stepchildren were in the home, compared with 87% of the natural and 72% of the adopted children. It is worth noting here that a child may leave home and return to the parental home several times before a final departure. Thus, because these data are right-censored, it is difficult to estimate whether or not children (especially those in their teens and early 20s) had actually left home for good. In fact, because of right-censoring, it is almost impossible to compare rates of leaving home for various age groups in any meaningful way. It appears that for most families (those with two to five children), the last child left home when the parents were in their early 50s.

The level of education attained by respondents was related to various family events (see Table 6.6). Divorce appeared to be curvilinearly related to education, in that those with either low or high levels of education had lower rates of divorce than those with moderate levels of education. Low levels of education were also related to being widowed, but this was probably so because education is an important dimension of

TABLE 6.6. Various Indicators of Marriage and Family Life by Educational Level, Canada, 1984

Indicator	Level of education					
	All levels	8 years or less	Some secondary	Secondary graduate	Some post-secondary	Post-secondary graduate
Of ever-married persons, percentage ever divorced						
All ages	11.3	9.2	12.3	13.1	11.3	9.2
Ages 30–39	13.7	12.3	15.2	17.2	13.4	8.4
Of ever-married persons 50 years and over, percentage ever widowed	12.4	15.3	10.9	11.1	11.5	. . .[a]
Of ever-married persons, percentage with two or more marriages	6.9	6.8	6.9	7.8	7.4	4.7
Of all persons, percentage ever in a common-law union						
Ages 30–39	21.1	15.8	21.6	23.2	22.3	19.5
Ages 18–29	23.4	29.1	30.3	20.8	20.2	23.1
Of all persons, percentage who have raised:						
Stepchildren	3.2	3.7	3.6	3.2	3.1	2.1
Adopted children	2.6	3.1	2.9	2.4	2.0	2.4
Of all women, percentage who have ever worked outside home						
All ages	86.2	72.0	84.1	90.5	89.8	95.1
Ages 30–39	93.4	77.7	90.7	97.5	96.8	96.7
Of women who have ever worked, percentage with one or more work interruptions	57.9	71.0	66.7	53.0	52.1	47.0
Of women with one work interruption, percentage reporting due to:						
Child care	42.3	28.4	36.9	49.4	48.6	50.4
Marriage	15.9	24.5	19.6	14.4	9.2	. . .[a]

Note. From *Family History Survey* (Statistics Canada, Catalogue No. 99-955) by T. K. Burch, 1985, August, Ottawa: Statistics Canada. Copyright 1985 by the Minister of Supply and Services, Canada. Reprinted by permission.

[a]Due to a high standard error, these figures are not shown.

TABLE 6.7. Reasons for Work Interruption among Respondents with One Interruption: Percentage Distribution Within Age Groups, by Sex, Canada, 1984

Sex and age group	Total	Marriage	Pregnancy or child care	Move to be with partner	Illness or disability	Layoff	Retire-ment	Return to school	Other and multiple reasons	Not stated
Male										
18–29	100.0	—	. . .[a]	. . .[a]	. . .[a]	54.4	. . .[a]	28.5	10.5	. . .[a]
30–39	100.0	—	. . .[a]	. . .[a]	14.1	37.9	. . .[a]	29.3	16.5	. . .[a]
40–49	100.0	. . .[a]	—	—	18.9	28.6	. . .[a]	27.2	21.9	. . .[a]
50–64	100.0	—	—	. . .[a]	27.0	20.7	22.6	8.0	21.1	. . .[a]
All ages	100.0	0.2[b]	0.3[b]	0.2[b]	15.6	36.5	7.0	22.4	16.9	0.9[b]
Female										
18–29	100.0	4.0	38.0	7.8	6.0	18.4	. . .[a]	10.1	14.8	. . .[a]
30–39	100.0	8.4	54.8	7.9	3.2	9.1	—	4.5	11.6	. . .[a]
40–49	100.0	20.9	47.4	5.5	6.1	6.1	. . .[a]	. . .[a]	8.6	. . .[a]
50–64	100.0	29.2	28.1	3.2	12.8	6.5	7.0	. . .[a]	11.7	. . .[a]
All ages	100.0	15.9	42.3	6.1	7.1	9.7	2.2	4.3	11.7	0.7[b]

Note: From *Family History Survey* (Statistics Canada, Catalogue No. 99-955) by T. K. Burch, 1985, August, Ottawa: Statistics Canada. Copyright 1985 by the Minister of Supply and Services, Canada. Reprinted by permission.

[a]Due to a high standard error, these figures are not shown.

[b]These percentages represent very few cases and therefore may contain a high level of error.

TABLE 6.8. Various Indicators of Marriage and Family Life by Province or Region, Canada, 1984

Indicator	Canada	Atlantic provinces	Quebec	Ontario	Prairie provinces	British Columbia
Of ever-married persons percentage ever divorced						
Ages 50 and over	9.2	6.5[a]	5.0	10.1	10.2	15.9
Ages 30–39	13.7	8.9	9.7	15.2	15.0	19.9
Of ever-married persons 50 years and over, percentage ever widowed	12.4	11.1	12.4	11.7	12.4	16.0
Of ever-married persons, percentage with two or more marriages	6.9	4.5	3.4	8.1	7.4	12.0
Of all persons, percentage ever in a common-law union						
Ages 50 and over	5.9	. . .[b]	5.3	6.7	5.6	7.2
Ages 18–29	23.4	16.6	28.3	19.1	24.7	29.0
Of all persons, percentage who have raised:						
Stepchildren	3.2	2.6	1.7	3.7	3.3	5.6
Adopted children	2.6	3.6	1.9	2.6	3.3	2.1
Of all women, percentage who have ever worked outside home						
Ages 50 and over	81.6	72.3	76.1	84.8	82.4	89.2
Ages 18–29	82.3	73.8	76.7	86.4	87.3	81.9
Of all women who have ever worked, percentage with one or more work interruptions	57.9	59.6	61.5	53.9	57.1	62.5
Of women with one work interruption, percentage reporting due to:						
Child care	42.3	41.2	35.0	47.4	42.2	45.1
Marriage	15.9	16.4	23.5	9.1	16.0	17.6

Note. From *Family History Survey* (Statistics Canada, Catalogue No. 99-955) by T. K. Burch, 1985, August, Ottawa: Statistics Canada. Copyright 1985 by the Minister of Supply and Services, Canada. Reprinted by permission.

[a]This percentage represents very few cases and therefore may contain a high level of error.

[b]Due to a high standard error, this figure is not shown.

socioeconomic status, and those in lower socioeconomic groups experienced higher mortality in general than those in higher socioeconomic groups. Education was also related to the percentage of women working outside the home. Table 6.6 shows that those women who had completed secondary school or attained higher education were more likely to have worked outside the home.

The Family History Survey also collected information on the respondents' history of work interruptions. Work interruptions were significantly related to family career, as can be seen from Table 6.7. Females were more likely to report a work interruption of at least 1 year in duration (49.9%) than were males (18.2%). Table 6.7 shows that the major reason for females' reporting at least one such interruption was pregnancy or child care, whereas for males the most frequently cited reason for such interruptions was being laid off. Clearly, for females, family career had an effect on their work career.

There were regional differences in the frequency of many family events. Table 6.8 shows that divorce varied by province, with British Columbia having twice as many divorces as Quebec and the Atlantic provinces. It is somewhat surprising to find that Quebec, which is over 80% Catholic, had such a high frequency of cohabitations for the younger cohort (28.3%).

To sum up, the Family History Survey supports the picture that Canadian families are more stable than their counterparts in the United States. Historically, Canadian divorce rates have been about half to two-thirds those of the United States. Cohabitation seems to be more popular with the younger cohorts, but it is still far from widely accepted as an alternative to marriage; only 5–6% of those surveyed were in a cohabiting relationship at the time of the study. The frequency of divorce varies by both region of the country and the level of education attained. Most Canadians see their children leave home when the parents are in their early 50s. With increased longevity and more stable marriages, this means that Canadians experience longer marriages than their counterparts in the United States and that a large proportion of their family life is spent in marriage without the children at home (Rodgers & Witney, 1981).

THE FAMILY STRUCTURE AND FAMILY CAREER PROJECT

With the assistance of Roy H. Rodgers, I designed and administered the Family Structure and Family Career Project. The design of the study was retrospective. However, some items, such as those from a marital satisfaction scale and interpersonal perception measures, were point-in-time measures rather than retrospective questions. The questionnaire was divided into four parts: a demographic section, a family event history section, the marital satisfaction scale, and questions regarding respondents' perception of their spouses' attitudes. The major differences between this study's design and that of the Statistics Canada Family History Survey were (1) that this project contained nonretrospective attitudinal measures, and (2) that though the sampling unit was the household, data were collected for both the husband and wife when possible. Thus, the principal unit of observation was the couple rather than the individual.

Couple data are often difficult to collect, and the Family Structure and Family Career Project did not escape these difficulties. One problem is that it is often difficult to obtain the cooperation of both individuals in a relationship. Another difficulty is the feeling that data on each individual will reveal dimensions of the relationship the respondents would rather not reveal. These problems may be responsible in part for the lower response rates and higher refusal rates for this type of data collection.

We attempted to address the many problems with collecting data on couples in the design of the study. First, the questionnaire format was kept as simple and time-efficient as possible. Second, knowing that refusals and nonresponses would be a major problem, we chose to use a strategy of increasing the sample size rather than intensively trying to recruit couples; thus, we mailed out questionnaires rather than conducting interviews. We realized that, regardless of the method of data collection, refusals would make the sample nonrandom. Furthermore, since there would be no sampling frame or list with couples rather than individuals, we decided to use the household as the sampling unit. Clearly, a random sample of households did not imply that a random sample of couples would be the result. We concluded that if we were going to have a nonrandom sample, it would be better to have one with a large number of cases (such as would be afforded by mailed questionnaires) rather than one with a small number of cases (such as would be afforded with interviews). Third, we felt that collecting what should be similar demographic data for two individuals in a relationship, as well as many family events that should be identical, would facilitate the assessment of the reliability of the responses in this type of design. Thus, we attempted to assure the quality of the data along with the quantity.

A questionnaire was mailed to approximately 3,000 randomly selected households in the Greater Vancouver Regional District (GVRD). The GVRD contains about a million and a half people. The simple random sample was selected from the 1983 phone directory on the first day of its public availability. The mailing was complete 1 month later, and all responses were received between June and August 1983. There were 1,059 usable returned questionnaires. This means that the study had a low response rate of about 35%. Although return rates of between 40% and 60% are usual for mail questionnaires, the return rate for this study was particularly low. This low response rate can be explained by two factors. First, when a household contained a married couple, the spouses were asked to fill out separate questionnaires, thus doubling the time and inconvenience. Another aspect of this is that in studies such as this one, when one questionnaire is sent to each household, it is usually the wife who completes and returns it; husbands are typically less willing to participate. Therefore, the statement that gathering couple data is doubling the difficulty is actually a conservative rather than a liberal estimate. The second factor affecting return rates was that of the nature of the information sought by the study. Other studies' average return rates are perhaps inflated by the fact that the areas surveyed are less personal and controversial. In this case, the sensitive areas of perceptual accuracy in the couple and the questions regarding marital satisfaction may have seemed too probing or of too intimate a nature; in other words, the sensitivity of these areas may have served as a deterrent to the return of the questionnaires. If these factors are taken into consideration, then the return rate does not appear too far out of line with those of other such studies.

Although there were 1,059 usable questionnaires, not all of these were received from people currently living with their spouses. People were asked to complete the part of the questionnaire pertaining to family career history even if they were currently single, separated, widowed, or divorced. In addition, some married persons returned their questionnaires without those of their spouses. When all of these were excluded, there were 313 couples or 626 married people in the sample with completed paired responses. This is clearly a smaller subset of the larger sample. There is the chance that this subset of couples may not have accurately represented the larger population of couples in the GVRD or in the province of British Columbia. It is therefore desirable to compare this subset of couples with those respondents in the Family History Survey who were currently married or cohabiting and living in the province of British Columbia. This comparison gives some idea of the extent to which this nonrandom sample was similar to the larger population from which it was drawn.

Table 6.9 shows that the couple sample from the Family Structure and Family Career Project contained a higher proportion of cases

TABLE 6.9. Comparison of Ages of Married and Cohabiting Individuals for Two Samples of British Columbians

	Couple sample		Family History Survey (weighted data)	
Age (years)	Male (%)	Female (%)	Male (%)	Female (%)
18–25	7.0	12.1	17.1	22.0
26–35	33.5	38.0	32.9	34.1
36–45	27.2	23.3	21.4	19.3
46–55	14.1	11.8	18.4	13.3
56–65	10.5	10.2	10.2	11.3
Over 65	7.3	4.5	n/a	n/a
Missing	0.3	—	—	—

between the ages of 26 and 45 than did the Family History Survey sample for the province. The largest difference for these age categories (26–45) was about 6%. There was a much greater difference between the two samples for the youngest age group (18–25): The percentages for the couple sample were 10% below the percentages found in the Family History Survey. Clearly, this group of young married people and cohabitors was underrepresented in the couple sample, whereas the age range 26–45 was overrepresented. These differences would seem to indicate that the couples in the couple sample were older and perhaps more stable than the general population of the province. Part of this difference may have been due to the different populations from which these samples were drawn. The Family History Survey sample was drawn from the province as a whole, whereas the couple sample was drawn from the urban area of Vancouver. Usually the age at marriage for couples is younger in rural areas, so this difference may in fact reflect a real difference between the two samples, rather than indicating that the couple sample was nonrepresentative.

Table 6.10 largely reflects the age difference in the two samples. Because the Family History Survey contained a greater proportion of young couples, it is not surprising to find that it also had a higher percentage without any children. That is, we might expect that these young marrieds were not having children yet. The higher proportion with one and two children in the couple sample reflects the urban character of the sample, in that smaller families are historically associated with more urban areas. As family size increases, the difference between the two samples reflects the more rural character of the Family History Survey.

TABLE 6.10. Comparison of Number of Children of Married and Cohabiting Individuals for Two Samples of British Columbians

Number of children	Couple sample		Family History Survey (weighted data)	
	Male (%)	Female (%)	Male (%)	Female (%)
None	23.3	26.2	30.1	30.2
One	19.5	18.2	14.9	14.7
Two	31.9	31.3	26.2	27.2
Three	14.7	15.0	15.2	15.7
Four	7.7	6.4	8.1	6.4
Five	1.3	1.6	2.6	2.8
Six	0.6	0.3	1.4	0.8
Seven or more	0.9	0.9	0.6	1.2

In other areas where comparisons are possible, these tend to support the contention that differences between the two samples do not indicate that the couple sample was unrepresentative of the Vancouver population from which it was drawn; rather, the differences seem to be due to the fact that the Family History Survey contained both urban and rural cases. For example, in the Family History Survey sample of the province, about 66% of both males and females had no postsecondary education; by contrast, in the couple sample, 54.3% of the males and 63.2% of the females had no postsecondary education. The higher education level of the couple sample again probably reflects the exclusively urban character of the population from which the sample was drawn. However, if these differences do reflect a systematic bias in the couple sample, it is clear that this bias was in the direction of better-educated, slightly older couples with two to three children.

CONCLUSION

This chapter introduces the two data sets to be used for subsequent analyses. Since the analyses require particular subsets of data from one or the other of the sets introduced, further comments are often required to characterize these subsets; therefore, the reader will have other opportunities to learn more about various descriptive aspects of these data as analyses proceed. However, it should be born in mind that subsequent analyses are aimed at illuminating parts of the theory of family development, rather than at making generalizations about some population. The concern here is with the generalizability of the theory rather than the generalization of empirical findings. Since well-developed theories can specify both the important variables and the boundary conditions under which they operate, we can assume that if the sample fits the boundary conditions, then the premises of the theory can be examined with that sample, regardless of the sample's representativeness of some particular population at a particular point in time.

ACKNOWLEDGMENT

The Family Structure and Family Career Project was supported by grants from both the University of British Columbia and the Social Sciences and Humanities Research Council of Canada (Grant No. 410-82-0733).

NOTE

1. For a full discussion of the complex methodology of the Labour Force Survey, readers should consult the Statistics Canada (1976) publication *Methodology of the Canadian Labour Force Survey*.

CHAPTER 7

The Process of Development: The Markov and Semi-Markov Assumptions

CHANGE, EVOLUTION, AND DEVELOPMENT

That families develop and change over time is a noncontroversial fact. What is of interest is the identification of patterns of change common to families. More particularly, it is of great interest to identify what changes in families are part of their maturation and development as organized social groups. A family is a social group organized around the tasks of reproduction, socialization, and kinship. As members of the group age and mature, the family changes. These changes are what theory of family development seeks to understand.

There have been many attempts to address the nature of development. Some of these attempts have sought to define development as a teleological process. But such attempts are doomed to failure unless one is willing to assume a metaphysical stance that is atypical of scientific inquiry. Other definitions of development have sought to define development as ontogenetic, in the sense that the genetic endowment of the organism contains and dictates the process of development. Such ontogenetic views are simply inappropriate for the study of development in social groups, because the group processes are as much a consequence of social-institutional norms that generate social structure as they are the summation of individual processes. Indeed, the process of development for a social group such as the family is a process composed of individual, group, and institutional effects. This process of family development includes the individual's maturation, the changes of the individual's roles contingent on the changes in another family member, and the changing institutional norms as they affect the social group of the family.

The process of family development is difficult to define. At a minimum, it can be characterized as a form of change. Three principal forms of change are relevant to families: "random change," "developmental change," and "evolutionary change." Random change is the most easily identified of the three; it is simply change in which the probability of an event or state is given by the frequency of the event's occurrence over time. Another way of expressing this is to say that any conditional probability is the same as the simple frequency of occurrence, and hence adds no information about the event.

Evolutionary change is actually composed of two types of change: change due to genetic material (e.g., mutations), and change due to natural selection's limiting a gene pool or population (Brooks & Wiley, 1986). Genetic change is characterized as linear and irreversible, in that changes move in the direction of greater specialization and cannot be undone. Natural selection, on the other hand, is a type of change in which adaptation to the environment limits gene populations. Whereas genetic change occurs within the individual organism, natural selection occurs at the level of the population. Since natural selection is contingent upon environmental changes, it is a form of change exogenous to the organism or population. That is, this type of change is not contained within the organism, as is the case with genetic change.

Developmental change is a process composed of effects from three levels: the individual, the social group, and the institution. It is a complex process and therefore, difficult to define. It includes effects that are both intra- and interindividual, intra- and intergroup, and intra- and interinstitutional. The only way to define such a process as family *development* is at the population or aggregate level. Although individual families may change and evolve and develop, the only way in which it is possible to isolate these various processes is by identifying the patterns at the aggregate level.

It is at the aggregate level that patterns emerge. Clearly, any one family could be studied over time, but it would not be possible to separate change from evolution or development. Only with several cohorts of families studied over time can these processes be identified in any meaningful way as patterns. Thus, it seems that a definition of the process of family development should focus on the type of patterns generated at the aggregate level.

The process of family development is defined as one in which a change of state is conditional on the duration of time in the current state. This definition assumes that development is a process in which time in a state may shift probabilities for possible subsequent states. This means that a family's immediate configuration of roles, norms, and internal relationships would determine the probabilities for the next stage of the family—that is, for the next configuration of roles, norms, and relationships. Furthermore, this definition assumes that the duration in a state determines the probabilities for the possible states. In other words, a family may be in a state or stage for 3 years, and up until that time the probability of state B as the next state may be .99. However, if the family is in that state for more than 3 years, the probability of the next state's being state B may drop to .25 and the probability of some other state Q may become .75. The probability is thus determined not only by the current state, but by the duration of time in the current state.

There are clear differences between this view of development and views of change and evolution. Genetic change, as noted above, is linear and irreversible, whereas in development probabilities may reverse, depending on the duration of time in a given state. Natural selection depends on the environment and is thus exogenous to the unit of analysis. However, development is dependent on the state occupied by the organism or family. This state is defined as an internal configuration (roles, norms, and relationships) that is characteristically different from the conditions brought about by natural selection. Change, in its broadest sense of random change, is different from this view of development, since in random change conditional probabilities are no different from the unconditional frequency of occurrence.

Although there are fairly clear differences among the processes of change, evolution, and development, some other processes cannot be so easily distinguished. The process of aging for an individual is similar to genetic evolution, in that it can be assumed that this process is monotonic and irreversible. That is, it is difficult to imagine someone becoming younger as time passes.

Experience as a process may be confused with development. "Experience" means the sum total of a family's or individual's states or stages (history or biography). This sum of experience might be expressed as a conditional probability that changes nonmonotonically with each new additional experience. This view of experience is very similar to that of development. The one difference between development and experience is that developmental processes show conditional probabilities based only on the time spent in the current state, whereas experiential processes show conditional probabilities based on a total sequence of states. With experiential processes, the Markov assumption that probabilities are at most dependent on the previous state would be violated. Thus, the major difference between experience and development is that development is defined as Markovian, whereas experience is not.

To sum up this discussion, family development as one form of developmental process is based on two assumptions. The first of these is the Markov assumption that the probability for moving to a state is determined by the current state. The second is the semi-Markov assumption that the duration of time in the current state determines the probabilities for the possible transitions. These two assumptions are the core of the process of development. Experience, evolution (both genetic and natural selection), and random change differ in significant ways from this view of development.

HYPOTHESIS AND ALTERNATIVE MODELS

Families change developmentally. This type of change is different from experiential change, evolutionary change, and random change. Family development is a different form of change because the process is a time-dependent Markovian process. The semi-Markov model discussed in the previous chapters makes this assumption. This chapter presents a test of this assumption and the competing models of change.

The model of change proposed by the semi-Markov model contains two testable assumptions: (1) that the probability of a move to another state is based on the current state (the Markov assumption); and (2) that the probability of a move is dependent on the duration of time in the current state (the semi-Markov assumption).

An alternative view of family change is the "experiential" view. This view actually contains two different models of change. One model is that the probability of a transition is based on the sum of all the past states experienced by the family or individual. For example, a family experiencing the sequence of events (states) in one particular order, such as marriage, birth, and divorce, would have a different set of probabilities for possible states than the family experiencing a different order of the same events, such as birth, marriage, and divorce. The semi-Markov model of development would claim that the set of probabilities is only conditional on the length of time each of these families has spent in the present stage of "divorced," and is not contingent on the previous sequence of stages.

A second model generated by the experiential view is that of the "efficacious event." This is the view that at some point in a family's history a particular event occurs that effectively propels that family toward certain transitions rather than others. For instance, one such event may be premarital births. The developmental model would suppose that the duration of time spent in the stage of "out-of-wedlock parents" determines the stage immediately following, but not later stages. The experiential view would assume that this event has an effect on later stages and not just those adjacent in time. Thus, the second model associated with the experiential view is that an event occurring at any point in the past determines the probabilities for the set of possible transitions.[1]

Another competing model for change in families is the "random change" model. This model assumes that the probability of any transition is simply given by the frequency of transitions to a state and that this transition is independent of past events. In this case, our theoretical perspectives on experience and development would not result in more accurate prediction of transitions, as would be the case with conditional probabilities. In this sense, the random change model simply confirms a state of ignorance about the process of family change.

METHODS

There are difficulties in testing these hypotheses. The principal difficulty resides in the problem that retrospective or longitudinal data on the family as the unit of analysis are virtually nonexistent. The individual remains the principal unit of analysis for most social science research. The only remedy to this state of affairs seems to be to use the individual's family history as a proxy for, or report of, family stages or events. The problem with this approach is that individuals' histories can be distinctly different from those of their families, as, for example, in the case of divorce, where one person gets custody of the children and the other person may go on to raise another family of procreation. Even with this problem, an individual's family history remains the best approximation of family event sequencing available.

A second methodological problem is the specification of a finite set of states or events. In order to test the hypotheses discussed above, it is necessary to have measures for the amount of time spent in a particular state and the transitions of all individuals to the next state. For one thing, the states involved must be relatively frequent for members of the population, so that sample size is not unduly restricted. Another consideration is that once the first state is specified, the possible transition states must be specified, so that the set of states is reasonably exhaustive and each state is mutually exclusive. As previously noted in Chapter 5, there seems to be no generally accepted theoretically determined set of states meeting these two criteria. This problem is compounded, in that the data to be used in this regard are data on events and not stages. Thus, a final problem is the specification of reasonable states by the events available in the data.

The beginning stages of family formation offer stages that both are relatively frequent in the population and can be linked to events in a noncontroversial way. A family is begun, by definition, when a child enters the scene. The event of the birth or adoption of the first child clearly delineates the transition to a family. This is true whether the parent is single, cohabiting, or married, since the definition of family is the presence of the parent–child, intergenerational bond.

The transition to a family may originate from several possible states. The individual may be single, divorced, widowed, married, or cohabiting. For present purposes we can lump single, widowed, and divorced into one category, which is designated here as "single." Thus, the states or stages prior to the arrival of the first child that are used in the present analysis are single, married, and cohabiting.

The hypotheses are that the longer one is married, single, or cohabiting, the probability of having a first child changes with this duration (the semi-Markov assumption of duration dependence), and that whether one is married, single, or cohabiting affects the probability of having a first child (the Markov assumption of state dependence). This second hypothesis may seem somewhat obvious, since we are all aware of the norms regarding childbirth out of wedlock. However, it is exactly this institutional aspect of family development that is being hypothesized here; furthermore, the emphasis is really upon duration dependence as a crucial element in family development.

The alternative hypotheses are several. First, there is the simple hypothesis that the process is independent of previous states. This hypothesis assumes that the probability of having a first child is the same as the conditional probabilities of having a first child if married, cohabiting, or single (random change model). A second alternative model is that of sequence dependence as proposed by the experiential view. This hypothesis would propose that there is some sequence of events that affects the probability of having a first child. Given the stages and events being used here, this hypothesis would suggest that those who have cohabited and then married have a different probability of having a first child other than that given by the duration in their present marriage. Yet another alternative hypothesis is the "efficacious event" experiential model, which proposes that some singular event determines the probability of having a first child, regardless of whether it is the preceding event or stage. This particular view might assume that those who have been previously divorced will have a probability different from that based on the duration in the adjacent state to the first child.

The data for this study come from the Family History Survey, described in Chapter 6. As I note in that chapter, I have assumed that the individual histories of the Family History Survey may be used as proxies for family histories. There are several limitations to this view. One is that individual histories report family events for individuals, not families. To assume that the individual history serves as a report on the history of the family is to assume mistakenly that the report is on the family unit, which it is not. Another problem with this assumption is that individuals get divorced and die, whereas the family unit, as defined by the parent–child bond, may continue to exist but may no longer be reported. In fact, those individuals who leave one family of procreation via divorce and then start another are clearly changing the family units in their reporting. Despite the limitations and faults of using individual family histories to represent families, this is probably the closest we will get until longitudinal data can be collected on family units over time.

The identification of the exact state or stage a survey respondent occupied immediately prior to the birth of the first child involves some difficulties. First, as noted above, there are a number of possible states from which a person can move to the birth of a child, including single, cohabiting, divorced, separated, and even "between cohabitations"! The initial step taken in this analysis is to compute the family careers for the following events: beginning first marriage, ending first marriage in separation or divorce, beginning first cohabitation, and ending first cohabitation. The same is done for events concerning the second marriage and second cohabitation. The order of events is computed by whether the birth occurred in the same year as listed for the beginning of the marriage or cohabitation, or prior to or during the year of the ending of the marriage or cohabitation.

The next step is to compute the duration of time spent in the state immediately prior to the birth of the first child. These time durations are only computed for the most interesting and frequent of states. Although individuals who have never married and never cohabited (i.e., who have always been single) are of interest to family scholars, there is no way to compute a duration in state for these cases, since there is no particular date at which the state of being single begins. So, in order to test the hypothesis concerning the duration of time in a state, only those states with a sizeable number of respondents and for which duration can be computed are used in the analysis.

RESULTS AND DISCUSSION

The Markov assumption suggests that the stage or state one is in prior to having a first child determines the probability of the likelihood of having a first child. With the strong social norms unfavorable to out-of-wedlock births, it is not surprising to find that the Markov assumption is supported in this case. Table 7.1 shows that over 83% of the survey respondents who were married made the transition to having a first child. The probabilities that respondents would make this transition from the states of single or cohabiting are rather small. Even when cohabitors are broken down into those who subsequently went on to marry their cohabiting partners and those who did not, the probability that they would have a child while cohabiting remains small (.04). Table 7.1 thus strongly supports the Markov assumption.

Table 7.1 also demonstrates the strong norms regulating mating and birth in North America. Outside of marriage, the next most likely state for the birth of a first child is being single. This is further evidence for the strength of the norms governing childbirth, in that many of these cases probably represent the youthful "mistakes" of respondents, since they had neither cohabited nor married.

One of the major threats to the Markov assumption is the "experience" explanation. This explanation views the state immediately preceding an event such as childbirth as being but part of a chain or sequence of events that explain or predict the birth. One way to test which of these two assumptions is most plausible is to compare the conditional probability based on the immediately preceding event to the probability based on a chain of events that contains as its last event the one used as the more simple preceding event. For example, the conditional probability of a birth in marriage can be compared with the conditional probabil-

TABLE 7.1. Probability of Having a First Child While Single, Married, or Cohabiting (n = 9,601)

State	Probability	n
Single	.105	1,008
Child prior to cohabiting or marriage	.088	(843)
Child during separations or divorce	.017	(165)
Married	.835	8,012
Cohabiting	.061	581
Later married cohabitant	.040	(387)
Did not marry cohabitant	.020	(194)

ity of a chain, such as cohabiting prior to marriage and then having a child.

Three states preceding the first birth are used in this analysis. The first state and the one occupied by the majority of respondents is that of marriage. Cohabitation is divided into two states: one in which the person was simply cohabiting immediately prior to the birth, and another in which the person cohabited, married, and then experienced the first birth. Using this last career allows a comparison of the conditional probability of simple adjacent states (the Markov assumption) with that of a history, as is implied by the notion of "experience." Thus, if "experience," or a longer chain of events does not yield a different conditional probability from that of the adjacent event, then the Markov assumption will receive additional support.

The probabilities of having a first child are quite different for those who were married and those who were cohabiting (see Table 7.2). However, the difference between those who were married and those who first cohabited and then married is relatively small (.049). This small difference is not a statistically significant one; it is also not theoretically significant, for several reasons. First, since cohabiting is still non-normative, there were undoubtedly a small number of respondents to the survey who did not report cohabiting. This would not be a large enough number to make up the difference between the cohabiting and married probabilities. A second reason is that cohabiting tends to be more popular among younger cohorts, and therefore some of these people might have children in the future but had not yet done so when surveyed. Thus, the right-censoring contains an age cohort bias that shows up in both higher rates of cohabitation for younger people and lower rates of childbirth, because they had not completed their fertility.

TABLE 7.2. Probability of Having a First Child in the Married, Cohabiting, and Cohabiting–Married States

State	Probability[a]
Married	8,012/10,472 = .765
Cohabiting	194/1,211 = .160
Cohabiting–married	387/540 = .716

[a]The probability is computed by dividing the number of those having a first child immediately adjacent to marriage (or cohabitation or cohabitation–marriage) by the total number at risk (e.g., all those ever married, ever cohabiting, or ever cohabiting–married). This analysis is restricted to first marriages and first cohabitors.

The importance of this argument regarding Table 7.2 is in terms of the hypothesis about "experience." One perspective on experience views it as a summation of past events. The hypothesis stemming from this view is that if "experience" makes a difference in explaining the birth of a first child, it should show a different conditional probability from the one that would simply be associated with the last state in the chain of experience. In relation to Table 7.2, the probabilities of having a first child in the married and in the cohabiting–married states should be different if the experiential hypothesis is true. However, since these probabilities are so close, it does not seem that the experiential explanation adds any information that is not already available from knowing the immediately preceding state. Thus, the Markov assumption appears the better alternative, at least in this particular case.

The second major hypothesis stemming from the semi-Markov model in regard to family formation is that the probability of a first child is determined by the duration of time spent in the state (the semi-Markov assumption).[2] This hypothesis gets at the essence of development. If family development means anything, it means that the duration of time spent in a state affects the probability of subsequent transitions, though perhaps not in a monotonic fashion. In the present case, the hypothesis is that the probability of having a first child changes with the length of time spent in a state (e.g., marriage).

Table 7.3 shows that people in each of the states previously examined spent different amounts of time in these states before having their first child. Cohabitors who had a first child spent the least amount of time between starting their cohabiting relationship and having their first child. As noted earlier, however, the probability that cohabitors would have a first child while cohabiting is fairly small. By contrast, the probability that married respondents would have a first child is much higher, but the married couples waited the longest mean average time before the birth (2.3 years). The analysis of variance does not directly address the hypothesis concerning the duration dependence of the prob-

TABLE 7.3. Analysis of Variance for Duration of Time in State Prior to the Birth of the First Child

State	Duration (days)
Married	856
Cohabiting	576
Cohabiting–married	728

Note. $F = 11.57$, $df = 2$, $p = .000$.

ability of having a first child, but does establish that the durations are different for these three groups.

The most interesting and theoretically important hypothesis is that the probability of the birth of the first child depends on the duration of time spent in a particular state. In order to test this assumption, the hazard functions of the groups must be compared. A "hazard rate" is defined as an estimate of the probability for a unit of time that individuals surviving to a time interval will not survive to the next time interval. The formal definition of the hazard rate is as follows:

$$\lambda_i = \frac{2q_i}{h_i(1 + p_i)} \qquad (1)$$

where λ = hazard rate for a given interval
q = proportion of terminal events
p = proportion surviving
h = interval width

This is simply to say that the rate is computed as the number of deaths (or whatever is defined as the terminal event) for each time interval, divided by the number of survivors at the midpoint of the interval. In the context of the present research question, the terminal event is the birth of the first child. Thus, the hazard rate examined here reflects the "hazard" of having a first child for each time unit.[3]

Figure 7.1 is a line graph of the hazard rates for each of the three groups analyzed above. The time interval is represented on the *x*-axis and is measured in 3-month units of 90 days. The entire time period covered in Figure 7.1 is the first 5 years of either marriage or cohabitation.

Although Figure 7.1 graphically displays differences in the hazard rates for the three groups, it is not possible to determine from this graph whether these differences are to be expected as random variation or whether there is systematic variation on the basis of the state or group. Table 7.4 shows the pairwise comparisons between these three groups, using the Lee and Desu (1972) *D* statistic. The comparisons in Table 7.4 test the null hypothesis that all subgroups or pairs are from the same survival distribution. The *D* statistic is based on a comparison of the individual's survival time in comparison with all other individuals in the sample. Each individual is assigned a score on the basis of increments or decrements of 1, when they survive or fail to survive another person. These scores are then weighted by subgroups and compared.[4]

Table 7.4 shows that although there are overall differences among the three groups, the differences between the pairs composed of those who were married and those who cohabited and then married are not statistically significant. However, there is a statistically significant differ-

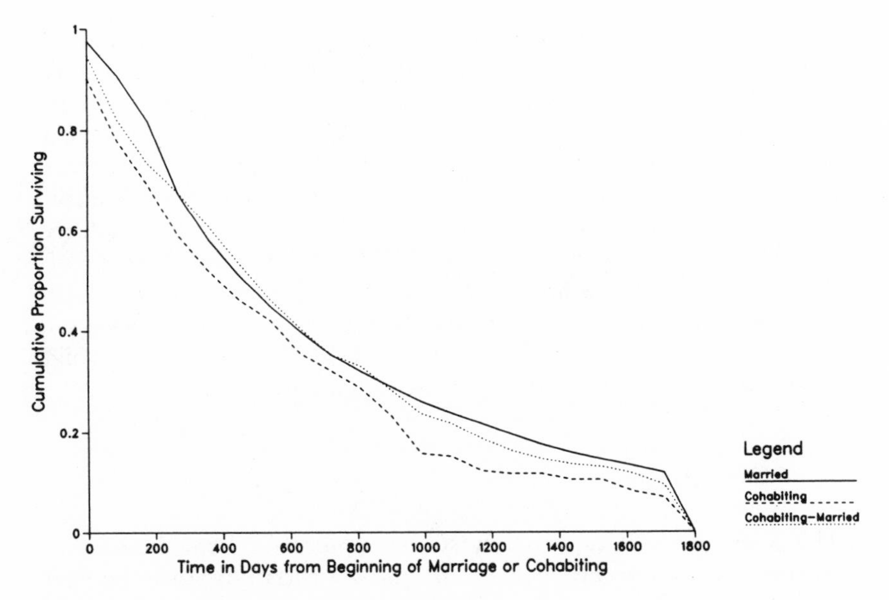

Figure 7.1. Hazard function for birth of first child.

ence ($p < .05$) between the survival function of those who cohabited and the function shared by those who were married and those who cohabited–married.

These findings suggest that within a state, the duration in the state affects the probability of the birth of the first child. This is support for the Featherman (1985) definition of development as duration-dependent. Furthermore, these data show that the duration in the state, and *not* the

TABLE 7.4. Overall and Pair Comparisons for Survival Rates (*D*) of Three States (Groups): Married, Cohabiting, and Cohabiting–married

States	Mean score	*D*	*df*	*p*
Married	39.3	11.46	2	.0032*
Cohabiting	–1,135.3			
Cohabiting–married	–309.6			
Married	24.0	9.90	1	.0017*
Cohabiting	–1,100.0			
Married	15.3	1.82	1	.1770
Cohabiting–married	–326.1			
Cohabiting	–35.3	3.23	1	.0722
Cohabiting–married	16.44			

* $p < .05$ (statistically significant).

history or experience, is what conditions the probability for a first child. If the history or experience were operating to determine the probability, then there should be a statistically significant difference between the hazards for being married and that for cohabiting and then marrying. Such a statistically significant difference does not exist in this analysis, and the conclusion is that these two groups are from the same survival function. The cohabitors, on the other hand, are probably from a different survival distribution, as predicted by the assumptions of the theory. That is, the theory assumes that both the immediately preceding state (the Markov assumption) and the duration in the state (the semi-Markov assumption) are related to the probability of the birth of the first child. These data support these theoretical assumptions.

CONCLUSION

This analysis provides relatively strong support for both the Markov assumption of state dependence and the semi-Markov assumption of duration dependence of transitions. These data clearly do not support the hypothesis that transitions are distributed at random. Otherwise, transitions would occur at the same rates and with similar probabilities, regardless of state. The evidence also casts doubt on the notion of "experience," where the meaning is the effect of the sum of all events experienced. If the experiential hypothesis were true, then there would be a difference between the probabilities of the married group and the cohabiting–married group. No such difference exists: The rates for these two groups are not statistically or theoretically different. This finding implies that only the preceding state and the duration of that state determine transitions.

The present analysis, however, has several limitations. First, at least one meaning of "experience" has not been tested—namely, the "efficacious event" meaning. It is quite plausible that marriage is such an event and that the present results could be used to support the view that throughout family life this one event of marriage is predictive of future transitions. Such a perspective, though possible, is not probable; the vast majority of people get married, but there are many distinct family careers, all of which include marriage. Thus, it seems unlikely that such a pervasive event is going to explain the variation in state transitions. For this reason, the interpretation of experience in terms of a single efficacious event does not seem to provide a fruitful avenue to explanation, even though it has gone untested in the current analysis.

Second, even though the interpretation of "experience" as a sequence of events has been examined in this analysis, the examination is severely limited. That is, it has examined the experience of only one event (cohabitation) prior to marriage. This is such a short event sequence that it may not reveal the effects associated with longer sequences of events. This point is worthy of some considerable digression.

The theory of family development defines "development" as a process in which transitions are both state- and duration-dependent. To say that transitions are sequence-dependent would be to contradict the Markov assumption of state dependence. However, the theory also states that if people or families do not follow the timing and sequencing norms, they are thrown out of synchrony with the age-graded institutions in their society, and hence are negatively sanctioned by missing out on life chances afforded to those who follow these norms. This statement regarding sequencing and timing norms implies that the probability of certain later states will change, depending on the timing and order of events sequenced. Such a perspective appears at odds with the Markov assumption that the dependence of transitions is only on the present state. The way out of this seeming contradiction is to distinguish between the effects on transition probabilities that are indeed Markovian (developmental) and the effects that are social-structural sanctions for deviance. This is to say that families at the aggregate level operate developmentally in regard to transitions, and that at the institutional level norms regulate and sanction the timing and sequencing of events. Thus, it becomes possible to examine family development at the aggregate level and to investigate family conformity and deviance at the institutional level of analysis. This distinction is further discussed in the chapters that follow.

The limitations of this analysis do warrant caution in the interpretation. It is not incautious, however, to say that these results suggest that family formation is a process whereby the probability of having a first child depends on both the present state and the duration of time spent in that state. For the presently married, the chances are very good for having a first child, especially in the first 3 years. For those presently cohabiting, the chances of having a first child are much lower, but the chances are that the child will come in the first 2 years of cohabiting.

Caution is most needed when examining the theoretical implications of these results. The random or null hypothesis appears very unlikely and can be rejected with some confidence. Also, the "efficacious event" hypothesis, though not directly tested here, nonetheless appears unlikely in relation to marriage and later career variation. Sequence dependence is not supported by these results, though any rejection of this hypothesis must be infused with a good bit of skepticism, since such a limited operationalization of sequencing is employed. The results thus most strongly, though not unequivocally, support the theoretical assumptions of the theory of family development that the process is both state-dependent and duration-dependent.

NOTES

1. Note that this model may also be compatible with the linear monotonic model and the natural selection model.

2. See Teachman and Polonko (1984) for a discussion of timing in the transition to Parenthood.

3. The following statistical analysis and parameter estimation were performed using the SPSS survival program. Readers should consult SPSS documentation for details (Hull & Nie, 1979). For a more in-depth treatment of the hazard function see Tuma and Hannan (1984), pp. 57–65.

4. For more detail readers should consult Hull and Nie (1979), pp. 29–30, or Lee and Desu (1972).

CHAPTER 8

Developmental Processes in the Couple

This chapter examines the process of development in the dyad. The dyad, especially the marital dyad, represents one of the most important and most researched of all the various family subgroups or relationships. The empirical research presented in this chapter does not add much that is different from the stable body of empirical knowledge about marriage (White, 1988). What is important in this chapter is the way in which old empirical research questions are reformulated into theoretical questions. Thus, the purpose of this chapter is to further develop the theory of family development in terms of family relationships and to illustrate these propositions empirically.

In regard to family subgroups, an important methodological and theoretical question arises: "What is the relationship between the individuals in a dyad and the dyad?" This question poses the problem of forming a group score out of some aggregation of individual scores. This is an area of some controversy. The basic position argued here is that only with comparative scores such as agreement or consensus can social-psychological constructs indicate the state of the dyad. All other types of social-psychological constructs (e.g., marital satisfaction) must be viewed as an individual's report on his or her subjective state, rather than as a report on the dyad. In cases where an individual is asked to report on the state of his or her relationship, that report should be treated like any other observation and analyzed for reliability with other reports, such as that from the other spouse. In this instance, we cannot hold out much hope for spouses having reliable assessments of the state of their relationships, since they often diagree in their assessments (e.g., Larson, 1974; White, 1985). Thus, the use of aggregated scores is suspect. Only the comparative analysis of individual scores at all approximates an indicator for the dyad. The preferred measures in regard to the dyad are qualitative measures of the state of the dyad and quantitative measures of the duration of time in the dyadic state. These measures not only are appropriate for the level of analysis, but are consistent with the theory of family development.

That the marital dyad is the focus of much scholarly activity is undeniable. However, much of this activity is directed at the individuals in the dyad rather than at the dyad itself. For example, one major area of scholarly attention is "marital quality" (Lewis & Spanier, 1979). However, the measures used in this area are typically measurements of the individual's adjustment, happiness, or marital satisfaction. These measures reflect the "personological" bias often encountered in family research (e.g., Featherman, 1985). That is, the individual and his or her internal states or processes are often viewed by researchers as "real," while other units of analysis (such as the dyad and the family group) are viewed as less "real" and more abstract constructs. Although there have been active discussions of dyads—as, for example, in discussions about the quality of the marital relationship—there exist few measures aimed at the dyad as the unit of analysis rather than the individual. By extension, much of the research on marriage is not about the dyadic relationship, but about the individual's perception of or report on the relationship. For instance, Anderson, Russell, and Schumm (1983) have reported that marital satisfaction is related to stages of the family in a curvilinear fashion. It is interesting that these authors do not draw greater attention to the fact that their sample was composed solely of wives. Thus, what their research has actually yielded is the wives' subjective marital satisfaction across stages of the family. It would be more theoretically appropriate to have research on the dyadic "quality" over time.

The dyad is a subsystem of the family, as is any other subgroup (e.g., triads). The various dyads in the family, such as the marital dyad, sibling dyads, and parent–child dyads, are all affected by the processes experienced by the family as a whole. However, each dyad has its own development, events, and stages. There exists little theoretical work identifying these stages and events for the various family dyads (and even less for triads), with one partial but notable exception. That exception is the marital dyad. (See Caplow, 1968, for an analysis of triads.)

The marital dyad is of great theoretical interest to scholars. Of all the dyads in the family unit, the marital dyad is the major unit formed by affinal rather than consanguineal bonds. Affinal relationships hold the possibility of choice; however, the choice of a mate is not always the preference of the future spouse, but may sometimes reflect the prescriptions of elders or the clan, or a tribal taboo (Lévi-Strauss, 1949).

Even in social systems where preferential mating is the rule, such as North America, there are formal constraints on who may marry whom. These are often codified in the legal system as "restricted degrees of consanguinity," although many of the restrictions forbid mating with nonconsanguines, such as a dead sister's husband or a dead brother's wife.

These codes or laws regarding mate selection serve to remind us that marriage is not simply a matter of love, intimacy, or sexual attraction between two individuals. Rather, marriage is a social institution as much as is the family. Marriage as a social institution is constructed of norms regulating whom one may marry, how one marries, and what the social roles of husband and wife (as well as the in-law relationships) include. Of course, not all of the many norms related to marriage are formalized in law. Many others are informal norms, such as those regarding division of labor. Sometimes it is surprising how many areas of marriage are covered, at least in part, by formal norms. For example, the areas of support and maintenance, ownership and property, and inheritance and descent are all regulated by at least a few formal and codified norms.

As a social institution, marriage is also regulated by timing and sequencing norms similar (and at times identical) to those regulating the family. The rope-jumping rhyme "First comes love, then comes marriage, then comes Suzie with a baby carriage" reflects timing and sequencing norms and the way in which they are learned by children. For example, the romantic love referred to in the rhyme is the event in North American culture regarded as the minimum sufficient condition for marriage. Furthermore, marriage is viewed as the institutional step that precedes having a family. Clearly, these norms establish a normative sequencing pattern and, when tied to the age- and stage-grading of the events, establish timing norms.

POSITIONS, NORMS, AND ROLES

The institutional nature of marriage provides the broad normative parameters within which each marital dyad functions. In order to understand how these institutional norms constrain and structure the marital dyad, it is necessary to recall the microgroup analysis in the theory of family development. This microgroup analysis is most clearly stated by Rodgers (1973). However, at the outset of this discussion, it should be noted that the present discussion gives a different meaning to the term "position" from that used by Rodgers. Otherwise, there is considerable agreement between these two formulations.

The term "position," in Rodgers's analysis, refers to "all the roles which belong together" (1973, p. 17). Rodgers's use of the term is critically different from the one provided here. "Position," as used here, means an analytic point in a social structure. This is to say that a position may exist independently of a role. As a concept, "position" is similar to "point" in geometry. A position can be defined for any abstract social structure, regardless of the real existence of that social structure in any society. Positions must be defined independently of roles in order to make cross-cultural research possible. For example, a "husband" is a position defined as "a married male." So the minimal social structure for this position is one distinguishing only gender and formalized affinity. Using this definition of the position of "husband," cross-cultural research can fill in the norms or expectations that are attached to this position (i.e., that constitute the role) in various societies. It is quite possible that the norms attached to this position are entirely different from culture to culture. Furthermore, this meaning of "position" makes possible the formal analysis of social structure (e.g., H. C. White, 1963) in the area of the family. Finally, it is consistent with the meaning used by Gross, Mason, and McEachern (1958), who define a position as a "location of an actor or a class of actors in a system of social relationships" (p. 48).

The term "norm" refers to a social rule that forbids, permits, or requires an act for a given position in a social system. Thus, norms are attached to positions, since positions are points in a social structure that may stand for classes of actors. Norms are what give the analytic point of a position its content. When all the norms for a given position are accumulated, the result is the social "role" for that position. For example, when for any given culture such as North America, all the norms are listed for a position such as "husband," the result is the role of husband. This role may contain norms forbidding adultery, permitting housework, and requiring maintenance of the family. The extent of an incumbent's ability to meet these norms is the incumbent's role performance.

Time is essential in the theory of family development. As families and family subgroups such as the dyad develop over time, they go through stages. Each stage is qualitatively distinct, in that its structure (positions and relations between positions) may change and the normative content may change. Clearly, the normative content and the structure interact. For example, if a father of a young family dies, the structure of the family changes. Attendant with this change in structure is a change in the norms regarding the mother's role. She is more likely to assume some of the expectations (norms) associated with the father's role. Since stages are defined by various structures and by the norms attached to the positions in the structures, the roles too must change over time. Hence, the norms that constitute the role of father for a very young family are different from the norms that constitute the role of father for an "empty nest" family. The important point in this regard is that the norms and roles change with transitions from one stage to another, but that the transitions are predicted by the present stage and by the duration of time spent in the stage. Undoubtedly, the duration of time spent in a stage varies with role performance as well as with forces exogenous to the family.

The dyadic positions in the family are the sibling dyad(s), containing brother and sister relations; the parent–child dyads, containing (1) father and son or daughter and (2) mother and son or daughter; and the marital dyad, containing husband and wife positions. At each stage, the normative content or roles for these positions change. These changes are governed by the timing and sequencing norms that establish the normative sequence for the various stages of the family. Thus, some role changes in the dyad are explained by the norms of the next highest system, the family. When the family changes stages, the roles within the dyads change.

To sum up this brief discussion, there are several dimensions on which the family as a microsystem or family subgroups such as dyads and triads may be examined. Most basic to any analysis is an examination of the positions and relations between positions, and the ways in which these change over time. This is the same thing as an analysis of the subgroup or group structure over time, since structure is given by the positions and relations between positions. A second dimension is the examination of the norms attached to any one position and the ways in which these change over time. A third dimension is the analysis of the roles of subgroups (dyads, triads, etc.) over time. The last dimension is the examination of the family roles over time. In all of these analyses, it must be remembered that the timing and sequencing norms regulating the most probable structures, norms, and roles are not analyzable from this microanalytic perspective, but only at an institutional level. That is, the rules governing the content of the norms and the process are given by the institutions of the family and marriage, and are not to any large extent generated by the individual family. Thus, to focus on the microanalytic level alone would leave scholars without the explanatory power afforded by the institutional norms. This is not to say that some changes in family dyads cannot be explained by dyadic developmental processes, but that a more fully developed explanation would include the institutional norms regulating the timing and sequencing of family stages, which serve as the context for the dyad.

STAGES OF THE MARITAL DYAD

The topic of developmental stages of the dyad is an extremely difficult one. In part, these difficulties are caused by the confusion regarding levels of analysis. At the individual level of analysis, stages are experienced as events in the individual's life course. At the dyadic level of analysis, stages are defined as shifts in roles resulting in changing patterns of interaction inside the dyad. At the group or family level of analysis, stages are defined by the structure of the family and the role relationships. As previously noted in other chapters, stages are not easily identified, nor do the existing stage systems meet minimal logical standards such as being exhaustive and exclusive.

Stages must be defined by the sequencing and timing norms that govern the processual development of the dyad. In other words, if there are stages of the marital dyad, then there must necessarily be timing and sequencing norms that are identifiable components of the *institution* of marriage. When we examine the norms regulating timing and sequencing of marriage, about all we find in this regard are processual norms related to family formation. It does not appear that there are any institutionalized sequencing and timing norms that apply to childless marriages; they apply only to those marriages that are moving to family formation.

This does not mean that childless marriages do not go through stages, but that these stages are not defined institutionally except when the marriage is a precursor of the family. Childless marital stages are not defined by institutional sequencing and timing norms; rather, marital stages of the childless are constructed from the interaction patterns in the dyad. When the marital dyad is part of a family, then these interaction patterns are constrained by the timing and sequencing norms of the family institution. But, in the case of childless marriages, there are no institutional timing and sequencing norms to constrain the interaction. Rather, the only normative constraint on the interaction patterns is given by the social norms regulating all marriages, such as those governing adultery and division of labor. These are static norms rather than processual norms. (The question of stages in childless marriages is discussed further below.)

Even those dyads within the context of the family and family stages go through their own transitions. So, although the family may be in a given stage, a dyad may go through several stages during this family stage. These dyadic stages are formed by interactions; however, they are constrained by the institutionalized family norms regulating sequencing and timing of stages. The process of development for these interactionally defined dyadic stages is the same as for family stages. That is, the process is characterized by state dependence and duration dependence: The probability of a transition is dependent upon the present state and the length of time spent in that state. As previously suggested, the relationship between the duration in a stage and the probability of a transition need not be monotonic. In fact, there are some states (e.g., marriage without children) in which, after a certain time in the stage, it is unlikely that a transition (in this case, to having children) will occur. This is not to say that the dyad may not keep developing. In fact, one area where our ignorance is readily apparent is in the identification of interactional stages for the marital dyad other than those based on family formation.

It is possible to outline the broad theoretical characteristics of stages for the marital dyad when that dyad is in the context of the family. At the structural level, the positions of husband and wife remain constant; thus, the structure of marriage is invariant. At the level of roles, it is clear that the normative content of these two positions change over time. Since the norms attached to the positions define the roles, it is a simple deduction to say that the roles change over time. A marital stage is defined as a qualitatively distinct period in the life course of the marital dyad. There are several transition points that are rather obvious disjunctions with previous norms and roles. For instance, when a child enters the scene, the marital roles are accorded a lower priority than they were previously, because the husband and wife must accommodate the new and demanding roles of father and mother. This change in family structure interacts with the normative content of the roles in the dyad. When the children leave home, the norms regulating the marital relationship suggest that it should regain the importance as an intimate and vital relationship it previously enjoyed. However, in a good many cases, a marital dyad is habituated to the parental roles and cannot successfully return to the norms that favor the marital dyad as the most important relationship. For example, many such awkward transitions are indicated by the husband's and wife's continuing to address each other as "Mother" and "Father" long after the last child has departed. Once their offspring have children, the grandparental roles are added to the marital roles; however, the marital roles are expected to remain the most salient to the aging spouses, since they will spend increasing amounts of time together. The couples who have maintained the parental roles and failed to return to the marital roles as most salient undoubtedly welcome the grandparental roles and let this role become central rather than the marital roles. Thus, the marital stages are largely defined by family transitions rather than by changes generated from within the dyad. These stages would, at a minumum, include early marriage without children, marriage with children in the domicile, late marriage without children in the domicile, and late marriage with grandparental roles.

Much of the research on the topic of marital satisfaction over stages of the family life cycle uses stages defined in a similar fashion to the ones in the preceding paragraph. However, the research in this area abounds with different sets of stages. For instance, Rollins and Feldman (1970) used a set of eight stages in their study of marital satisfaction, whereas Anderson et al. (1983), in a test of the U-shaped curvilinear relationship between stages of the family life cycle and marital satisfaction, used only five stages. As previously noted, there is no set of theoretical stages commonly attributed to the development of the marital dyad, and this confusion is reflected in the empirical work. The characterization of stages (not events) offered above is simply one among a large number of possible sets of stages for the study of marriage. The major problem with all of these is that they rely on the fact that most marriages lead to families, and have developed their stages on the assumption that marriage is the institutional precursor of the family.

An alternate way of approaching the development of the marital dyad is not to attempt identification of theoretical states, since this has also proven difficult in regard to family development. Rather, the approach could be to identify important dyadic events that are commonly regarded as transition points. So, for example, marriage, remarriage, separation, divorce, cohabitation, ending a cohabiting relationship, and death of a spouse or cohabitant are all dyadic events of great significance. Thus, without identification of the states that these indicate, it may be possible to agree on the importance of these events as transition points and to analyze some of the theoretical assumptions using these indicators. However, this is only a methodological sidestepping of the theoretical problem of identifying truly dyadic, interactional stages of development. Furthermore, with an event approach to dyadic transitions, the unit of analysis is typically the individual's experience of transitions into or out of a type of dyad. Hence, events such as divorce and separation are transitions out of the dyad, and events such as beginning cohabitation or remarriage are transitions into the dyad. This is a far cry from the identification of dyadic states based on interaction patterns. The event approach relies heavily on the institutional norms governing marriage, which, as previously noted, are not sequencing or timing norms but static norms.

One question that requires an answer at this juncture is "What are the stages for marriages that remain childless?" The answer seems simple at first. Marriage is an institution that is established by timing and sequencing norms as a precursor to family. There are undoubtedly stages to childless marriages, but such stages are developed from interaction patterns between the husband and wife and between the couple and the environment. These stages are not products of the institutional norms, since the institutional norms are almost totally oriented to marriage as a beginning point for a family. Of course, the formal norms regulating marriage, such as those governing maintenance and property, apply to all marriages, but these formal norms are not processual. The event approach is one of the few that provides categories relevant to marriage dyads both within and without families.

The research on dyads is not sufficiently developed to identify the stages of the childless marriage at this time. In the last 10 or so years, many researchers (e.g., Gottman, 1979) have focused on the identification of states formed by interaction patterns. There have also been some formal attempts at delineating interactional stages (White, 1982). However, at this time, none of these are sufficiently well formulated as microtheories of developmental stages in the marital dyad to be integrated into the theory of development.

These approaches are in general characterized by their focus on the dyad as a system of "mutual contingencies." Farber (1961) describes the family as a set of mutually contingent careers. This notion of mutual contingencies makes especially good sense in relation to interactional stages of the marital dyad. The marital dyad moves through stages such that the state of one individual is contingent upon the state of the other. This suggests that the individual level of analysis is important in analyzing the dyad. For instance, a husband's individual state is contingent on his wife's individual state. These contingencies may be immediate in time, but are much more likely to be lagged, so that person B's response to person A's action is a delayed response. The dyadic stage is marked by the types (patterns) and direction of these contingencies. One reason this area has not been further developed theoretically is that much of the empirical research is couched in a behaviorist perspective, which affords little impetus to develop theory (e.g., Gottman, 1979; Gottman & Porterfield, 1987; Noller, 1984).

MUTUALLY CONTINGENT PERSPECTIVES

The marital dyad is sometimes mistakenly characterized as a set of "complementary" roles. In the marital dyad, as in all family dyads, the roles are sometimes defined in a complementary fashion: Sometimes what is required of one spouse is forbidden to the other. But it is also often the case that relations are noncomplementary (e.g., adultery is forbidden to both). It is therefore inappropriate to characterize marital roles in general as complementary. The behavioral approach used to study interaction patterns avoids this pitfall. However, the lure of a simple description of the marital dyad as "complementary" still exists. The description of the dyad as a "mutually contingent" relationship avoids this mistake and seems more appropriate.

One area, besides the behavioral, where the perspective of mutual contingency in marriage is used with some frequency is the area of interpersonal perception scores. Researchers from diverse backgrounds have found this an attractive approach to the analysis of marriages and other dyads. For example, Kelley and his associates (1983) in psychology; Niemi (1974) in political science; Larson (1974) in sociology; and Laing, Phillipson, and Lee (1966) in psychiatry have found variants of this approach useful. The connection with the notion of marriage as a mutually contingent relationship is quite clear: If the contingency exists between two people, then what person A thinks about an issue and what person B thinks about the same issue should be related. That is, a husband's perception of the world should be related to the wife's perception of the world, and vice versa. McLain and Weigert (1979) refer to the process by which spouses come to share the same world view as a process of "biographical fusion." As spouses share the same stance in the world and the same experiences, their perspectives on the world become more nearly similar. Thus, spouses' perspectives are mutually contingent, in that the perspective of one spouse should predict with some accuracy the perception of the other.

In the area of marriage and the family there is a considerable history of research examining the perceptual differences between spouses (e.g., Dymond, 1954). For example, many early studies on mate selection (e.g., Kirkpatrick & Hobart, 1954) examined the proposition that those with similar perspectives are more likely to wed. Laing et al. (1966) tied together what was previously a rather disparate group of research methods into a coherent methodology. These authors identified several levels at which dyadic comparisons of individual perceptions can be made. Their work is important in the area of the family because it is one of the few attempts to link the individual level of analysis with the dyadic level without recourse to some arbitrary aggregation of scores. In fact, what Laing et al. pointed out is that the comparisons are ones many of us use in our everyday lives as members of dyads.

The two comparisons that are most often used are what Laing et al. (1966) termed "agreement" and "understanding." Basically, these two comparisons are created as difference scores between the perceptions of individual spouses for a specific issue. For example, if a husband and wife are asked the question "Do you want to have children?" independently of each other, then the comparison of their answers as a difference score indicates "agreement" if there is no difference. That is, agreement is indicated if both say "Yes" or both say "No." Of course, the question may be rephrased into a statement with a Likert-type response scale for finer gradations of agreement. What is important here is the truly dyadic or group nature of the construct. That is, agreement (or what some prefer to call "consensus") is a property of dyads and groups, and not an individual property except in the most trivial sense of self-consistency.

The second dyadic comparison is "understanding." This construct means that one person accurately knows the other person's view, regardless of whether or not he or she agrees with or shares that perspective. So, for example, the following question, linked with the response to the question above, provides a difference measure for understanding: "Does your spouse want to have children?" If we compare the husband's response to this question with the wife's response to the question regarding whether or not she wants children, the result as a difference score indicates that the husband understands his wife if there is no difference. However, this measure lacks the same dyadic property that agreement has, because the understanding is possessed by an individual rather than being the property of the dyad. Either the husband understands his wife or the wife understands her husband, but it takes an aggregation of the individual understanding scores in order to say that this is an "understanding" relationship. This same problem applies to the higher levels of comparison identified by Laing et al. (1966). The problem with these measures is that they are definitely based on dyadic comparisons, but in order for the construct to make any sense, the measure must be attributed to the accuracy of the individual's perception rather than to a property of the dyad. Thus, the comparison of understanding involves a somewhat ambiguous interpretation, since it is both dyadic in one sense and individual in another sense. The comparison of agreement, however, measures a dyadic or group property (i.e., consensus) and stands as an unambiguous dyadic measure.

It is illuminating to contrast agreement as a dyadic measure with the more often used measure of "marital satisfaction." Marital satisfaction measures are based on individual responses alone. These responses are seldom matched between spouses so that the differences between husbands' and wives' scores on marital satisfaction can be examined. Often, only one gender is used to respond, as in the Anderson et al. (1983) study. These difficulties can often be resolved by collecting data on couples rather than individuals in couples. Then, even individual marital satisfaction scores can be used to construct an agreement score for the dyad on marital satisfaction or any single item or dimension. The problem with sampling couples rather than individuals is that there is seldom a sampling frame for couples; as a result, this type of research must often sacrifice a considerable degree of representativeness for the study of the relationships within the sample. Thus, what is lost in external validity is traded off for greater internal validity.

To sum up, this discussion of the marital dyad emphasizes three points. First, the marital dyad goes through the same developmental processes as does the family. These processes are state dependence and duration dependence. The major stumbling block to the analysis of the development of the marital dyad is that no set of stages has been identified for the marital dyad as a unit independent of the family. This problem is most acutely brought into focus when we consider that the application of family stages to the marital dyad leaves the childless couple with few if any stages, since most of the stage conceptions are based on the presence of children. One way around this problem is to use an event approach to the study of development in the marital dyad.

Second, the discussion thus far in this chapter suggests that nonfamily stages for the marital dyad are probably defined by the couple's interaction. In the long run, interactional research may provide some delineation of these stages, but at the present time this is not the case. However, the idea that marital interaction can be characterized in terms of the mutually contingent perspectives of spouses suggests that dyadic measures such as "agreement" or "consensus" can be used to measure the couple's interactional state. If we reason that interactional states are related to couple event transitions, then dyadic consensus or agreement should change with the event measures of state and duration. Thus, it is possible to further explore the notion that dyadic interaction is a developmental process.

Third, the vast majority of research on the marital dyad focuses on measures of marital satisfaction, marital adjustment, or marital happiness, or what Lewis and Spanier (1979) call "marital quality." Marital quality is a subjective measure of how happy or satisfied one spouse is with the marital relationship. Although this is an *individual*-level measure, one cannot help asking how subjective marital quality is related to dyadic development.

HYPOTHESES

The theoretical discussion has highlighted several problems with researching development in the dyad. It is impossible to offer a definitive examination of the process at this point in the maturation of the theory.

However, the foregoing discussion suggests three areas in which empirical explorations might shed some light on the process of dyadic development.

The principal hypothesis in regard to stages is that duration of time in a stage and the present stage determine the probability of the next stage. Since no existing system of stages has been developed for the marital dyad, the next best approach in this regard is to specify events and the duration of time between events as indicators of stages. This skirts the theoretical problem of specifying the stages, and yet implies that the events used are in fact important transition points in the development of the marital dyad. The hypothesis in this regard (hypothesis 1) is that the duration of time in a stage is related to the probability of the transition to the next stage. In event terms, if the starting event is the beginning of cohabitation, the length of time spent cohabiting is related to whether the next event is marriage or the end of cohabiting. If the starting state is marriage, then the duration in this state is related to the chances of separation, divorce, and death of a spouse.

The next question is this: "Is the stage or duration in a stage related to dyadic scores?" In this regard, it is of great interest to find out whether duration in a state is related to dyadic differences in marital satisfaction scores, and to dyadic perceptual agreement scores (hypothesis 2). Is couple agreement contingent on the stage (as indicated by the most recent event) and the duration of time in that stage? From the existing empirical literature, we know that length of marriage, at least for wives, is related to marital satisfaction scores (e.g., Anderson et al., 1983). This, in addition to the theory, suggests that the duration of time in a state is related to dyadic consensus.

Lastly, there is this question: "What is the relationship between the events in dyadic development and the individual's perception of marital quality?" The hypothesis in this regard (hypothesis 3) is that the events used to infer dyadic stages and the duration of time in the stage are related to the individual's assessment of marital quality. This hypothesis is not derived from the theory so much as from curiosity, since the dependent variable is clearly at the individual level of analysis, whereas the independent variables are at the relationship level. However, it is interesting from the perspective that the relationship is both the context and object of such individual assessments.

METHODS

Data

The data used in this analysis are from the Family Structure and Family Career Project (1983), which surveyed 313 couples. As previously discussed in Chapter 6, this project was a retrospective survey that included marital and family event histories, in addition to a number of point-in-time measures. Among the point-in-time measures were a marital quality scale developed by Norton (1983) and several attitudinal items. The attitudinal items allowed the comparison of one spouse's responses with the other spouse's.

Marital Events

The present analysis is an event analysis rather than an analysis of stages. However, the definition of "event" (Allison, 1984) indicates that an event represents a relatively sharp disjunction between what precedes and what follows it. The definition implies that an event is a transition point between stages. Events are used to infer the model's construct of "state." The relationship between the model's construct of "state" and the theoretical concept of "stage" is supposed to be isomorphic. Because of the difficulties in identifying the theoretical stages, this issue is skirted for the moment. Such sidestepping is justified on the grounds that the theory of development has paid insufficient attention to the specification of stages for the marital dyad that are independent of the stages of the family. As discussed previously, the reason for this state of affairs is probably that timing and sequencing norms are derived from the institution of marriage and the family, and this institution treats marriage as a precursor to the family. Nonetheless, the marital dyad does change states over time, independently of the family sequencing and timing norms; however, these changes are interactionally based rather than normatively based. At a minimum, these changes of state are indicated by events that are commonly regarded as transition points. For instance, the birth of the first child is commonly regarded as a transition point between the stages of early marriage and the newly formed family, but this transition point is clearly relevant only to those dyads forming a family. More universal to the marital dyad are events such as death of a spouse, separation, remarriage, divorce, and the beginning or ending of cohabitation. These events are commonly regarded as transition points for the marital dyad.

The marital events used in the present study are identified from the respondents' chronological ordering of the following possible events:

Marriage
Remarriage
Death of spouse
Separation
Divorce

Reuniting with spouse
Beginning cohabitation
Ending cohabitation
Reuniting with cohabitant

The chronological ordering for these events represents each individual's marital career as opposed to the family career. The respondents also provided the date (year only) in which each event occurred. Although having only the year rather than the month and day provides a crude estimate of duration, there were no zero entries for duration, indicating that simultaneity at this level of measurement is not a problem for these data.

Individual Marital Quality

Marital quality was measured by Norton's (1983) Quality Marriage Index (QMI). All respondents who considered themselves as members of a couple living together, whether actually married or cohabiting, were asked to respond to the marital quality section of the questionnaire. There were 278 married couples and 35 cohabiting couples in the sample; however, the responses to the marital quality section are missing for some individuals and hence for some couples. For example, the first of the six QMI items shows two missing responses from cohabitors and four missing responses from married individuals.

The QMI is constructed from responses to six items. These items were found by Norton (1983) to be highly intercorrelated and, hence, were assumed to be measuring the same dimension. Norton has argued, contrary to Spanier (1976), that a marital satisfaction measure should be one-dimensional rather than multidimensional, and should leave other areas such as spousal communication and spousal affect as independent variables that might explain spousal satisfaction with the relationship. Since Norton's work, others have supported this type of approach to marital satisfaction (e.g., Fincham & Bradbury, 1987). The scores for each of the six items are transformed into normal scores, since the number of possible responses varies between items. These normal scores are then averaged across all six items. The mean QMI scores and standard deviations for males and females in the Family Structure and Family Career Project are reported in Table 8.1. These data support the unidimensionality of the scale, as well as its reliability (alpha for males' QMI = .917; alpha for females' QMI = .918).

The QMI results for husbands and wives are not significantly different, as can be seen from Table 8.1. These aggregated scores may conceal considerable differences at the couple level, since it is quite possible to have no difference in group means but to have a significant lack of correlation between the members of each pair or couple.

Dyadic Consensus

Dyadic agreement scores are constructed for two different areas.[1] First, a difference score is computed by subtracting the husband's QMI score from his wife's QMI score. Spousal agreement on marital satisfaction is indicated by a difference score of 0. The second difference score is computed as the average difference between husband and wife on seven issues. The spouses' perceptions on the seven issues are measured by the Likert-type responses to the following statements:

1. Children need strong physical discipline.
2. Leisure time should be spent with friends rather than family.
3. My spouse makes the greater financial contribution to the relationship.
4. I do most of the household chores.
5. One spouse gives more to the relationship than the other.
6. A woman should have the right to have an abortion without the consent of her husband.
7. A woman with preschool children should not work full-time.

The use of husband and wife difference scores would reveal little if marital agreement were the rule. However, as many authors (e.g., Larson, 1974; White, 1985) have pointed out, there is considerable difference between spouses on many issues. The issues used in this study support this finding. Table 8.2 shows the correlations between the husbands' and wives' perceptions on each of the seven issues. If there were agreement between the spouses, then the correlations would be both positive and strong. Note that this is not the case for these seven issues; the correlations in Table 8.2 are positive, but not strong. In fact, they are

TABLE 8.1. Description of Aggregated QMI Scores for Husbands and Wives

Variable	Mean	*SD*	Minimum	Maximum	*n*
Husbands' QMI	0.02	0.87	–0.50	4.70	303
Wives' QMI	0.02	0.99	–0.61	9.37	299

TABLE 8.2. Correlations between Husband's and Wife's Scores on Seven Issues

Issue	r
1. Discipline	.5711*
2. Leisure	.4067*
3. Finances	.5200*
4. Chores	.2348*
5. Gives more	.3111*
6. Abortion	.4494*
7. Working mothers	.5463*

*$p < .001$.

surprisingly low when one considers that spouses must share chores, leisure time, and family responsibilities. The fact that these coefficients are positive and statistically significant pales in importance when one considers, for example, that spouses in this sample agreed with each other on a woman's having an abortion without her husband's consent only about 20% of the time ($r^2 = .2019$). In order to place this in some perspective, the probability for agreement by chance alone if two individuals' responses are independent is .0625, or 6.25% of the time.

The issue statements cover a wide range of issues. Some of these issues may be more salient for some couples than others, depending on the stage of family life. Also, these issues cover a broad range of family activities and represent a multidimensional approach to perceptual agreement. Table 8.3 shows the lack of association of agreement on one issue with agreement on another issue.

TABLE 8.3. Correlations between Agreement (Difference) Scores for Spouses by Issue

	1. Discipline	2. Leisure	3. Finances	4. Chores	5. Gives more	6. Abortion	7. Working mothers
1.	1.00	.2536**	−.0476	.0970	.0494	−.0097	.1231
2.		1.00	.1125	.1120	.0705	.1845*	.1173
3.			1.00	.3299**	.0689	.2126**	.0642
4.				1.00	.1070	.1927**	.0174
5.					1.00	−.0075	.0544
6.						1.00	.0187

*$p < .01$.
**$p < .001$.

A principal-components analysis has identified three factors from these seven items. Factor 1 is composed of the items related to leisure, finance, chores, and abortion. Factor 2 consists mainly of the item related to discipline of children. Factor 3 is composed of the issue related to one spouse's giving more in the relationship. These factors are not used in the present analysis, for two reasons. First, the three factors do not account for 44% of the total variation in the pool of seven scores; therefore, use of the factors would fail to represent the total variation in the difference scores. Second, the use of an average of the absolute difference scores is a better and more readily interpretable measure, in part because it does not arbitrarily reduce the variation in scores. Variation is represented as the average difference on all seven items. This average score implicitly assumes that all items are of equal importance when averaged over all cases. This is not unreasonable. As I have noted, the salience of these seven issues probably changes with stage of the family; however, when the salience is averaged over all cases, it would be expected that it would approximate a random distribution. In other words, the number of people who find abortion the most salient issue should approach the number who find child discipline the most salient issue. This average of absolute differences across all seven issues is called the average perceptual difference score. It, like the difference score between husbands' and wives' QMI scores, is a dyadic-level score.

RESULTS AND DISCUSSION

Hypothesis 1

The hypothesis that dyads are subject to the same developmental processes that regulate families can be stated in the form of this question: "Are the dyadic stage transitions dependent on the stage and the duration of time in that stage?" This question is addressed here as one concerning these event transitions: marriage, separation, divorce, death of spouse, beginning cohabitation, and ending cohabitation. There are different transition matrices for husbands and wives. Often, it is the case that spouses share the same events, such as having cohabited together and subsequently married each other. However, it can also be the case that one spouse has cohabited several times and has previously married and divorced before marrying the present spouse, while the partner has not experienced any of these events.

The data show a small difference between the transition matrices of husbands and wives, created by the fact that three more of the males claimed they were married than did the females. Otherwise, the only major difference between the two matrices is that 10 more males than females had been previously married and separated.[2] This difference is due to the differences in age between husbands and wives. Table 8.4 shows the frequencies for transitions between these events for husbands, and Table 8.5 shows these frequencies for wives.

Tables 8.4 and 8.5 show that the patterns of transitions are distinctly different for the states indicated as pertaining to cohabiting and married couples. If we use Table 8.4 to illustrate these differences, one obvious difference is the institutional difference that events such as divorce only pertain to the institution of marriage. When we compare the percentage ending cohabitation (26.6%) and the percentage either separating or divorcing (19.8%), there appears more stability in marriage than in cohabitation. In addition, a far higher percentage continued in the married state (78.1%) than continued cohabiting (48.4%). However, if cohabitation is viewed as a developmental step toward marriage—and, in line with this reasoning, both those who continued to cohabit and those who married are viewed as continuing in stable relationships—then the percentage of those moving from cohabitation to a stable relationship at

TABLE 8.4. Husbands' Transition Matrix for Dyadic Events

	Time 2					
					Cohabitation	
Time 1	Marriage	Separation	Divorce	Spouse death	Cont.	End
Marriage (n = 247)	78.1% (193)	18.2% (45)	1.6% (4)	2.0% (5)		
Cohabitation (n = 64)	48.4% (31)				25% (16)	26.6% (17)

TABLE 8.5. Wives' Transition Matrix for Dyadic Events

	Time 2					
					Cohabitation	
Time 1	Marriage	Separation	Divorce	Spouse death	Cont.	End
Marriage (n = 244)	81.1% (198)	14.3% (35)	2.5% (6)	2.1% (5)		
Cohabitation (n = 67)	40.3% (27)				22.4% (15)	37.3% (25)

time 2 (73.4%) is very close to the percentage continuing in marriage (78.1%). On the other hand, if we examine dissolution rates, we find that cohabitations end with greater frequency than marriages end through divorce and separation. This suggests that whether a couple starts the marital career by cohabiting or getting married makes a difference in the stability of the relationship, but perhaps not as large a difference as might be guessed from an initial glance at Table 8.4 or Table 8.5. In regard to the effect of state on the transition probabilities, these data suggest that these probabilities are state-dependent.

The next question in regard to the developmental process is the question regarding duration dependence. Another way of stating this is that the probability of a transition depends not only on the state, but on the duration of time in that state. Table 8.6 shows the cell means for the duration of time males spent in each state (cohabitation or marriage) before making a transition to the next state. There are only minor and insignificant differences between males and females in regard to duration, so the data presented in Table 8.6 are approximate representations of the durations of relationships for both males and females.

Table 8.6 shows quite a difference in duration in state for those who were married rather than cohabiting at the beginning of their marital history. Cohabitors married about 1½ years after beginning cohabitation, whereas those who continued to cohabit had been cohabiting for about 3½ years. On average, those cohabitations that broke up did so after about 2½ years. On the other hand, it is quite clear that marriages lasted for a longer duration even when they ended in separation or divorce. Table 8.6 suggests not only that the state (cohabitation or marriage) affects which transitions are most probable, but that the duration of time in that state also clearly affects the transition ($F = 26.49$, $df = 6$, $p = .000$). This finding strongly suggests that the event transitions of dyads are subject to the same developmental processes as those of families.

TABLE 8.6. Duration (Years) in Marriage or Cohabitation before a Transition for Males

	Time 2					
					Cohabitation	
Time 1	Marriage	Separation	Divorce	Spouse death	Cont.	End
Marriage	19.71	7.76	13.5	22.8		
Cohabitation	1.52				3.47	2.41

Note. See text regarding the applicability of these data to females as well as males.

Hypothesis 2

The basic developmental hypothesis is that the probability of a transition to a state is dependent upon both the present state and the duration of time spent in the present state. This view of development naturally leads to the question of whether the dyadic measures vary in a similar way. However, state dependence and duration dependence must operate in a different way than they do in regard to the probability of a transition to another state. In this case, state dependence and duration dependence are viewed as explaining the variation in the dyadic scores for the difference in spousal marital quality and the difference in perceptual agreement.

In order to examine the effect of the present state and the duration in the present state on these dyadic measures, a two-way analysis of variance is used. Since the sampling unit is the couple rather than the individual, there are only two possible states, either marriage or cohabitation. The duration in state is divided into the following categories: 0–3 years, 4–5 years, 6–10 years, 11–20 years, and 21 or more years. The reason for using these categories rather than equal time intervals is that they represent relatively well-defined periods of social time. That is, in general, the first 3 years of marriage are usually a time of adjustment; the period of 4–5 years usually represents the addition of children; years 6–10 are the years in which couples most often divorce[3]; years 11–20 are usually stable for those marriages that have survived; and the period of 21 or more years usually represents the return to more couple-oriented activities with the departure of children (e.g., Rodgers & Witney, 1981). Some of these time periods make sense for cohabiting couples. Most cohabitations survive 1–3 years (White, 1987b), and thus fall within the first time period. Cohabitations lasting longer than 3 years are relatively unusual.

The dyadic score for differences between the husband's and wife's assessments of marital quality can reveal more about the relationship than the individual scores. The most important aspect of this dyadic difference score is that it represents paired observations, whereas individual mean scores lose this information. With aggregated individual scores, the only appropriate inferences are those concerning the individual. The dyadic measure moves us to the couple or relationship level of analysis.

The difference in spouses' assessments of marital quality vary by state ($F = 6.801$, $df = 1$, $p = .01$) and by the two-way interaction of state and duration in state ($F = 5.495$, $df = 3$, $p = .001$). A mean difference score of 0 would mean complete agreement between spouses' assessments of their marriage. Note that agreement between assessments of marriage is closest to 0 for relationships in the first 5 years and after 20 years. These data thus only partially support the hypothesis that dyadic interaction is developmental in nature. However, even this must be regarded as only a tentative conclusion, because the interaction effect must be regarded as suspect, given the small number of cases of cohabitors at different levels of duration. Table 8.7 shows the cell means for the interaction; the means for the main effects are shown as marginal means.

The dyadic average perceptual agreement scores are composed of the differences between husbands and wives on the seven items listed earlier (discipline, leisure time, etc.). The interpretation of these perceptual agreement scores is similar to that of dyadic differences in marital quality: A score of 0 reflects the same score for husband and wife, but does not tell anything about the direction of the attitude. The variance of the dyadic perceptual scores is also similar to that of the dyadic differences in marital quality. That is, perceptual agreement in couples varies by both state ($F = 3.795$, $df = 1$, $p = .052$) and the interaction of state and duration ($F = 3.819$, $df = 4$, $p = .005$). Table 8.8 presents the cell means for this relationship.

The effect for state on couples' agreement suggests that married couples agreed more closely on these seven issues than did cohabiting couples. This finding is interesting, especially in light of the previous finding that individuals in cohabiting relationships reported higher relationship quality assessments than did married individuals. The significant effect for the two-way interaction is certainly suspect in regard to Table 8.8, since the "6–10 years" cell for cohabitation has only five cases

TABLE 8.7. Cell Means for Differences in Marital Quality (QMI) between Spouses (Husband Minus Wife) by State and Duration in State

	State		
Duration	Marriage	Cohabitation	Main effect for duration
0–3 years	–0.02 (54)	–0.03 (19)	–0.02 (73)
4–5 years	–0.01 (25)	0.00 (1)	–0.01 (26)
6–10 years	–0.15 (39)	–1.91 (6)	–0.39 (45)
11–20 years	0.12 (62)	–0.42 (2)	0.10 (64)
21 or more years	–0.01 (84)	[a]	–0.01 (84)
Main effect for state	0.00 (264)	–0.46 (28)	

Note. n's for each cell are in parentheses.
[a]No couples in this cell.

TABLE 8.8. Cell Means for Dyadic Average Perceptual Difference Scores by State and Duration in State

	State	
Duration	Marriage	Cohabitation
0–3 years	0.32 (52)	0.32 (19)
4–5 years	0.35 (25)	0.36 (2)
6–10 years	0.33 (38)	1.11 (5)
11–20 years	0.28 (56)	0.21 (2)
21 or more years	0.34 (72)	0.43 (1)
Main effect for state	0.32 (243)	0.46 (29)

Note. Only significant ($p < .05$) main effects are reported. *n*'s for each cell are in parentheses.

and a score that must be regarded as an outlier. We can see from the cell means that if duration is important in regard to perceptual agreement, it is only so for the cohabiting couples and not for the married couples. The agreement scores for the married couples are relatively stable across the levels of duration. Thus, the major conclusion in regard to perceptual agreement in couples is that it varies only by state (marriage vs. cohabitation). As in the case of the data shown in Table 8.7, the two-way interaction must be regarded as tentative at best. It would be incautious to say that spousal agreement appears to be related to both state and duration. This final point must await confirmation from longitudinal research with a larger sample size.

Hypothesis 3

The major hypothesis examined in this section is that the dyadic stage and the duration of time in that stage are related to the individual's assessment of marital quality (hypothesis 3). Several ancillary questions emerge at this individual level of analysis. One of the first questions to arise is whether or not individual spouses' marital satisfaction scores (QMI) are related. A second question that arises in regard to the dependent measures is this: "Are the dyadic-level dependent measures (average perceptual difference and QMI difference scores) related to the individual-level marital quality (QMI) scores?"

Table 8.9 shows the association between dyadic scores and individual QMI scores. The table indicates that the perceptual differences for couples are not related to the husbands' assessment of marital quality, but are related to the wives' assessment of marital quality. This is

TABLE 8.9. Correlations between Dyadic and Individual Measures

	Individual QMI scores	
	Husbands	Wives
Dyadic scores		
Average perceptual difference	.0094	.4548*
QMI difference	.3474*	−.6624*
Individual scores		
Husbands' QMI		.4724*

*$p < .001$.

particularly important, since many measures of marital satisfaction (except for Norton's QMI) include agreement as one of the most important dimensions of marital satisfaction (e.g., the Dyadic Adjustment Scale). This finding suggests that this may be true for wives but not for husbands.

Table 8.9 also shows a relatively strong relationship between the QMI difference score and the individual QMI scores for spouses. However, there is a large artifactual component to the association, since the individual scores construct the dyadic difference score. Thus, a strong relationship between these variables is neither surprising nor of any substantive significance.

It is of much greater significance that the individual scores are associated. There is a moderate relationship between the husbands' assessment of marital quality and the wives' assessment of marital quality ($r = .4724$). This coefficient appears in quite a different perspective when interpreted as the variance explained ($r^2 = .2232$). This means that only about 22% of the time did husbands' QMI scores roughly agree with their wives' scores. Once again, it is surprising that spousal evaluations are not much more highly correlated.

Perhaps the most obvious question in regard to differences between spouses is whether or not those differences are due to some differences in individual characteristics that were present at the time of marriage. For example, it would not be unusual to expect spouses of different religions or from different cultural backgrounds to hold different perceptions about such issues as abortion and division of labor.

Correlations between the respondents' number of children, age, income, and education, and husbands' and wives' QMI and the perceptual difference scores, reveal only one statistically significant coefficient. This is the one between husbands' income and the dyadic measure of perceptual differences ($r = -.171$, $p < .01$). This finding suggests that as husbands' incomes increase, perceptual differences diminish. However, this finding is of marginal substantive significance, since the variation in husbands' income accounts for only about 3% of the variation in perceptual agreement scores.

The relationships of the dependent measures with religion and ethnicity are examined by a one-way analysis of variance. Neither husbands' nor wives' religion or ethnicity has a significant relation to the dependent measures of perceptual agreement, differences in QMI scores, husbands' QMI scores, or wives' QMI scores. Thus, the conclusion is that these variables do not account for variation in the dependent measures.

It seems an obvious extension of the present research to examine the relationship between state and duration for these individual scores, as has been done for the dyadic scores. The analysis of variance for husbands' QMI scores shows that neither the present state nor the duration in state has a significant main effect on husbands' assessments of marital quality. However, the two-way interaction of state and duration in state does have a significant effect ($F = 3.843$, $df = 3$, $p = .010$). This effect is shown by the cell means in Table 8.10. This interaction effect is similar to the others that have been previously discussed, and is suspect for the same reasons.

There are several points of interest in regard to Table 8.10. First, among those who are married, the husbands' QMI scores do not in any way resemble the U-shaped curve for marital satisfaction discussed by Rollins and Feldman (1970) and others since then (Anderson et al., 1983). Rather, the findings in Table 8.10 suggest that husbands assess marital quality as being relatively low during the early years. Second, during the

TABLE 8.10. Cell Means for Husbands' QMI Scores by State and Duration in State

	State	
Duration	Marriage	Cohabitation
0–3 years	–0.06 (54)	0.24 (21)
4–5 years	–0.07 (25)	1.87 (2)
6–10 years	0.10 (39)	–0.27 (7)
11–20 years	–0.08 (64)	–0.15 (2)
21 or more years	0.00 (88)	[a]

Note. Only significant ($p < .05$) main effects are reported. *n*'s for each cell are in parentheses.
[a]No subjects in this cell.

first 3 years of cohabiting, males appear to assess their relationships more favorably than males in the first 3 years of marriage. Comparing Table 8.10 to the dyadic differences for the QMI in Table 8.6, we see that the lowest scores for males on the QMI occur at the same time as the highest dyadic agreement. I have reported a similar finding elsewhere (White, 1987b).

The results for wives' marital quality assessments are somewhat different from those for the husbands' assessments. State ($F = 6.438$, $df = 1$, $p = .009$) and duration ($F = 2.272$, $df = 4$, $p = .048$) have significant main effects on wives' QMI scores. The two-way interaction of state and duration is not significant for wives, whereas it is significant for husbands. However, this interaction must once again be viewed with suspicion, because of the small number of cases in the cells for cohabitation by duration levels. Table 8.11 shows the significant main effects as the marginal means, and the interaction cell means are presented for comparison with those for husbands in Table 8.10.

The cell means for married wives by duration in Table 8.11 are similar to those for husbands though not statistically significant. For wives, state, independent of the duration of time spent in the state, has an effect on the assessment of the marriage: The QMI scores for cohabiting females are higher than those for their married counterparts. Duration in the relationship, independent of the type of relationship, also makes a significant difference in how the relationship is assessed. The first 3 years are more positive than for husbands, followed by a decline in assessed

TABLE 8.11. Cell Means for Wives' QMI Scores by State and Duration in State

	State		
Duration	Marriage	Cohabitation	Main effect for duration
0–3 years	−0.06 (56)	0.22 (20)	0.01 (76)
4–5 years	−0.08 (26)	−0.39 (1)	−0.09 (27)
6–10 years	0.23 (40)	1.67 (6)	0.42 (46)
11–20 years	−0.18 (62)	0.27 (2)	−0.17 (64)
21 or more years	−0.02 (85)	[a]	−0.02 (85)
Main effect for state	−0.03 (269)	0.50 (29)	

Note. Only significant ($p < .05$) main effects are reported. n's for each cell are in parentheses.
[a]No subjects in this cell.

marital quality during years 4–5. This decline reverses during years 6–10; assessed quality then falls again during years 11–20.

This complex pattern for assessed marital quality suggests some similarities for both spouses. It seems that female cohabitors report higher marital quality than married spouses. For both spouses, assessment of marital quality is highest during years 6 through 10. This is somewhat surprising, in light of the research on the U-shaped relationship between stage of the family life cycle and marital satisfaction. It is also surprising, given that these years are usually the ones with the highest rates of separation and divorce. One possible explanation of this finding is that these people are the survivors of relationship breakdown; hence, the poor-quality relationships may have been selected out of the sample, since the spouses in these relationships are no longer together. This explanation, however, leaves the unanswered question "Why does marital quality then fall in the subsequent duration?" Another possible explanation may be a sampling bias created by the self-selection of respondent spouses who both complete a questionnaire.

Comparing Table 8.7 with the tables for individual QMI scores (8.10 and 8.11) reveals some interesting differences. It must be kept in mind while examining these tables that the dyadic difference scores are interpreted as follows: A difference score of 0 indicates that two partners assessed their relationship in the same way. They may both have assessed it as low in marital quality or high in marital quality. So the difference scores in Table 8.7 measure agreement on the assessment, not the actual quality of the marriage. With this in mind, it is interesting to note that although individuals reported greater quality in cohabiting relationships, Table 8.7 shows significantly less agreement on couples' assessments of marital quality in cohabiting relationships as opposed to marriages. Table 8.7 suggests that on average, marital agreement on the quality of the marriage is the rule. Furthermore, the duration period of 6–10 years, which shows the greatest individual satisfaction with the relationship, also shows the greatest disagreement between married spouses on that assessment. The negative difference score indicates that a wife's assessment is generally higher than a husband's assessment during this duration period.

CONCLUSION

It is difficult to reach conclusions about developmental processes in the dyad from cross-sectional data. However, in this study, the data regarding transitions are the respondents' retrospective reports of their marital history. This form of retrospective data stands as a good approximation of a longitudinal design. The problem here is that many of the other dependent variables are measured as point-in-time or cross-sectional measures (QMI and perceptual difference scores). Therefore, conclusions regarding the effect of developmental processes on these particular dependent measures are constrained by this limitation in the data.

The dependent measure of marital quality (QMI) for males shows no relationship with married state or duration in that state. This suggests that males' perception of marital quality is not significantly affected by developmental processes; that is, their perception of marital quality is not a function of some set of temporal variables, such as duration or length of marriage. For females the picture suggested by these data is quite different. Female marital quality varies by marital state and duration, with cohabitors reporting greater marital quality than married women.

Dyadic differences in the assessment of marital quality vary by the couple's state (marriage vs. cohabitation) and by duration. For married couples, the years of greatest dyadic disagreement on the assessment of marital quality are years 6–10 of marriage. Yet these same years are the ones in which both spouses report the highest average marital quality. However, the wives tend to report higher marital quality than the husbands at this point, resulting in the significant difference between the two marital assessments for this time period. Indeed, married wives report greater highs and lows in their marital quality than husbands report. This is evidenced by the difference scores for marital quality for the time periods of 6–10 years and 11–20 years.

By contrast with the swings in the dyadic agreement on marital quality, the dyadic perceptual agreement is relatively stable over these time periods for married couples. However, though cohabitors report higher marital quality than married spouses, cohabitors have significantly lower perceptual agreement in their relationships. Agreement in marriage may well be tied to task coordination in marriage. The reason why cohabitors do not show the same degree of perceptual agreement as in marriage may be that there is greater individual rather than couple emphasis on problem solving. This emphasis on the individual versus the couple may in part explain why cohabiting females report higher marital quality than married females. If tasks require couple coordination, such coordination may also require greater effort to achieve consensus on issues. If cohabitors are more likely to respond to tasks as individuals rather than as a couple, then this may be conducive to maintaining a relatively conflict-free relationship, and may also require less personal energy. Furthermore, the great bulk of cohabitors are in the early years of the relationship, where some degree of idealization may exist. These cohabitors in the early years may also be viewing cohabitation as a prelude to marriage, and hence maintaining high subjective evaluations of the relationship.

All of these conclusions are subject to several limitations. First, it is inappropriate to assume that cross-sectional measures are in any way adequate to examine developmental processes. In this sense, the conclusions above are merely suggestive that such relationships *may* exist. Second, the small cell populations for various durations of cohabiting make any conclusions regarding state *and* duration impossible. Again, the data for the QMI and perceptual difference scores are merely suggestive at this point. What this analysis does indicate is that there are relationship-level measures that are suitable for the investigation of developmental processes at the relationship level of analysis, without recourse to the individual or family levels.

The hypothesis regarding the probabilities for a transition to another state (hypothesis 1) takes advantage of the retrospective design, and hence does not have the same severe limitations as the other hypotheses (2 and 3). Hypothesis 1—namely, that dyads are subject to the same developmental processes as families—is supported by these findings. Tables 8.4 and 8.5 show that transition probabilities shift significantly, depending on the starting state. This suggests that dyads exhibit state dependence. Table 8.6 shows that duration in the starting state has an effect on which transition state is most probable. These data suggest that duration dependence, as well as state dependence, characterizes dyadic transitions.

These results are based on retrospective accounts of marital history, and thus serve as an appropriate indicator for processual analysis. The results strongly suggest that dyadic transitions are developmental. However, all of the results may be explained by the competing hypothesis that they are due to dyadic maturation alone. It is virtually impossible to rule out this competing hypothesis, since duration in state, age, and length of time in the dyad are all related. That is, the problem of multicollinearity makes this question largely unresolvable. Although the competing hypothesis is viable, it and the developmental hypothesis are not mutually exclusive. That is, it is most likely that both individual maturation and dyadic development account for transitions. It does seem clear from these findings that a significant part of dyadic change appears developmental in nature.

The results of this study must be placed in the larger theoretical perspective. The states for the dyad are constructed from events that mark moving either into or out of a dyadic relationship. This is not the best imaginable way to construct dyadic states or stages. It would be preferable if interactional research were sufficiently well developed that states of the dyad could be identified from patterns of interaction or profiles of scores. At this time, this does not seem to be possible. But the states used in this study lack this interactional component. Indeed, the assumption in regard to the states used here is simply that moving into and out of a relationship implies the most basic dimension of interaction—that is, presence or absence. Although this is an incontrovertible dimension of relationships, it must also be considered rudimentary compared to potential interactional stage demarcations. So it remains an open question whether duration in an interactionally defined stage determines the probability of a transition to the next interactional stage.

The larger theoretical context for family dyads, whether marital, sibling, or parental, is afforded by the higher levels of analysis. A genuine understanding of dyadic development is only possible once the family and institutional norms are understood. For example, a marital dyad situated within a family structure with many members is likely to behave differently from one where no children are present. As we shall see, the stage of the dyad is linked to the stage of the family. Furthermore, each family stage contains a unique constellation of roles and norms. Some of these norms are static (within a stage) and some are processual. These norms and expectations for the future undoubtedly have an effect on marital, sibling, and parental dyads in ways unaddressed in this chapter. Although this chapter has attempted to examine the developmental processes in the marital dyad as an independent dimension, it is clear that the other levels of analysis may afford yet a deeper understanding of these family subsystems.

NOTES

1. The computation of difference scores is an area of some methodological debate and controversy. There are complex arguments for using raw difference scores, absolute difference scores, and various transformations of difference scores. In this work, I have stayed close to the raw scores, because they provide the sign or direction of difference between husbands and wives. In the computation of averages, the absolute scores are used. The reader is referred to the discussion by Cronbach (1958) for a discussion of most of these methodological issues.

2. Note that the small difference between husbands and wives here also gives considerable credibility to treating an individual's report of family events as a proxy for the family's career.

3. This is most true for the large recent Canadian marriage cohorts from 1960 to 1974 (Burch & Madan, 1986).

CHAPTER 9

Cross-Institutional Sequencing and Timing Norms

The previously described empirical investigations have laid the foundation for the present chapter. In Chapter 7, the investigation has suggested that both the family stage and the duration of time spent in that stage assist in determining the probability of transitions. In Chapter 8, the data have supported the view that dyadic change is developmental. The present chapter examines the proposition that institutionalized norms regulate the sequencing and timing of events. This perspective on family transitions views the probabilities as being determined by cross-institutional social rules or norms, which then are expressed in the sequencing of the normative careers of individuals, couples, and families. Thus, in this perspective, the duration of time in a state and the contingent path of a spouse are both regulated by these higher-level, institutional normative structures.

The present chapter investigates several dimensions of cross-institutional event sequencing and timing. The major theoretical construct employed here is that social norms from the institution of the family and other social institutions regulate the order of family events and the timing of those events. A lengthy discussion is needed to clear up some controversies about sequencing and timing norms, prior to the empirical examination of the effects of different event sequences. This discussion involves, first, a definition of sequencing and timing, and recognition of the problem that these two concepts are not independent. Second, the discussion deals with the perspective that family events are normatively regulated, and the recent critique of this perspective by Marini (1984).

The empirical section of this chapter demonstrates that different orderings for the same events are related to different consequences in later life. This seems to point out that indeed there are interinstitutional connections between life event sequences. The empirical investigations also show that the modal or most frequently occurring sequences have the lowest rates of disruptions in later life, regardless of the marriage cohort (length of marriage). It is important, however, to note that the norms for event sequencing are different for males and females, as are the effects for sequencing on work and marital disruptions.

DEFINITIONS

At the outset, it is important to note that the norms regulating event sequences and those regulating the timing of events are not independent. That is, both of these sets of norms really come from one relatively coherent body of age-graded and stage-graded norms. In fact, the order of events in the life course is just a crude way of measuring the timing of these events. However, this is not to say that important dimensions of timing and ordering cannot be conceptually distinguished.

The most basic conceptual distinction between norms regulating the timing of events and norms regulating the sequencing of events is that the sequencing norms say nothing about the age at which an event should occur, nor about the duration of time that should be spent in the stage. For example, the children's rhyme cited earlier in this book in no way suggests the length of time one should be married before having a child, nor does it specify the age at which one should have a child. It does, however, express the norms regarding the sequencing of events.

Two dimensions of timing norms have been identified by Featherman (1985) as "age-graded transitions" and "event transitions" (cf. Chapter 3). He points out that age-graded transitions are based on the chronological age of the person, as in most age-graded institutions (e.g., schools). Event transitions are based on the duration of time in a certain state, such as the length of time since the beginning of cancer and the probability of death. The problem with these two notions is that often they cannot be empirically separated, since both contain the same underlying dimension of time and both are usually highly correlated. For instance, the age at which one enters kindergarten is highly correlated with the amount of time spent in kindergarten. So, although these two can be conceptually distinguished, they are often empirically confounded.

Sequencing contains several dimensions as well. One dimension is what might be called the "event" dimension. This refers to the identification in a sequence of an event not shared by other sequences. For instance, cohabitation used to be a rather infrequent event or stage before marriage. When this was the case, two mate selection sequences such as

(1) dating, engagement, marriage and (2) dating, cohabitation, engagement, marriage would be difficult to assess as to the effect of ordering, because very few sequences would include cohabitation as an event. Thus, most studies of sequencing exclude this event dimension by only examining different orderings for the same states or events.

This immediately suggests the second and most researched dimension of sequencing, which is the order of the states or events. The ordering of events implies the comparison of the effects for different orders of the same events. For instance, one might compare marital satisfaction for (1) individuals with the order for early life events of marriage, first job, first child, and (2) individuals with the order of first child, marriage, first job. One problem that arises in such analyses is that time—in terms of both duration and age-grading—is involved in the analysis. In the example given here of event orders, pregnancy and childbirth clearly place more time constraints on starting a first job than does marriage. In this sense, some element of duration in state is involved in the comparison of orders. There is also an element of age-grading, since institutions such as work have minimum and maximum ages for employees and for certain types of work. Thus, for adolescents it may be easier to have children and get married than it is to have a job, because of the age-graded nature of work. The point here is that the study of sequencing or ordering of events is not independent of time or of timing norms.

The fact that time, duration of time in a state, chronological transitions, and the nature of the events are all tied together in the study of event sequencing is not that surprising. One implication of this is that when we are speaking of timing and sequencing norms, we must keep in mind that these norms are so interwoven as to represent one set of relatively coherent norms governing life event or stage transitions. Thus, norms governing the age at which one begins work also influence the timing of other events and the probability of various orders. In the present context, it is important that the implications of this confounding be expressed in terms of the limits on theoretical claims. For example, it is possible to speculate whether or not an effect is more closely related to chronological age than to duration in a state, but most often this is an empirically unresolvable issue.

SEQUENCING AND TIMING NORMS

Neugarten, Moore, and Lowe (1965) first suggested that there are age-graded norms regulating the timing and sequencing of life span events. This perspective is shared by a great many scholars studying the social structure of individual and family development (e.g., Elder, Hogan, Hill, Rodgers, and Aldous, to mention but a few). However, Marini (1984) criticizes this "normative model" of development and calls for its abandonment. Her criticisms are based largely on the understanding that social norms have sanctions attached to them. If in fact there are timing and sequencing norms, she argues that there should also be social sanctions for not following those norms. She points out that there is scant evidence that such sanctions exist, other than the exploratory work by Neugarten et al. (1965). Marini cites the work of Modell (1980), which suggests that in terms of timing, behavior changes occur prior to attitudinal changes. Marini sees this as evidence for the invalidity of frequency measures for social norms, since the behavior changes first and these changes are seemingly independent of the attitudes.

Marini's criticisms are serious ones, and yet they have received scant attention from developmental scholars. Hogan and Astone (1986) respond briefly that Marini confuses levels of analysis, but do not explore their rebuttal in sufficient depth. The major problem with Marini's critique is indeed her confusion regarding the different levels of analysis. However, this is a confusion shared by many scholars, even those who would oppose Marini's perspective. In order to understand Marini's confusion in regard to levels of analysis, we need first to re-examine the concept of "norm," and second to identify the appropriate constructs at each level of analysis.

Before the beginning of the substantive discussion, the terms "concept" and "construct" need to be clarified. There is a distinct difference between the two. The distinction made here follows that made by Kerlinger (1973). A concept is an abstraction expressed in either formal or natural language. For example, "norm" is a concept meaning a social rule regulating social behavior. A construct, on the other hand, is also an abstraction but is necessarily tied to a set of measures. For example, "IQ" is a construct with different dimensions, such as verbal and analytic ability. The concept that the construct is supposed to measure is "intelligence." Given the plethora of IQ tests available, it is clear that sometimes there are multiple constructs for a single concept such as intelligence. The same is true of the concept of social norms, with the additional caveat that different constructs are necessary for different levels of analysis.

The concept of "social norm" is, on the surface, a simple one. A norm is a social rule regulating social behavior. However, the concept of "norm" has received many different definitions from various social scientists. Not all of these definitions contain the same elements, nor are they necessarily consistent with one another. Rodgers (1973) returns to

Bates for his definition: "Bates (1956:314) has stated that a norm is 'a patterned or commonly held *behavior expectation*. A *learned response* [emphases added], held in common by members of a group' " (1973, p. 16). It is evident from this definition that there is some confusion as to whether norms refer to (1) the actor's cognitions (expectations) or (2) the actor's behavior (learned responses). Indeed, this ambiguity occurs throughout the vast literature on social norms, with scholars taking one side or the other, or maintaining that norms are both behavior and expectations.

The meaning of "norms" that this book uses is shared by many sociologists. It is the definition of norms as social rules. Bierstedt (1970) introduces this meaning with the example of a baseball game:

> [B]aseball, like other games, would be impossible without rules. These rules are norms, and one may say that they constitute the structure of every game, from baseball to bridge. We then looked up into the grandstand and noticed that the spectators were conforming to rules too. These rules are also norms, the norm appropriate to viewing a baseball game. . . . What is true of baseball in this respect is equally true of all the situations of society. Whatever order and regularity they exhibit is attributable to the presence of norms to which participants, in various degrees conform. A norm, then is a rule or standard that governs our conduct in the social situations in which we participate. (p. 209)

The seeming simplicity of this conception of norms conceals many dimensions. For instance, some scholars invariably use "expectations" as a synonym for "norms." Others believe that there are measurable sanctions attached to all norms (Gibbs, 1965). It has also been the case that the concept of "norm" has been discussed by many scholars as though it were appropriate for only one level of analysis. For example, the idea that norms are related to social approval or disapproval is restricted to the group level of analysis and largely inappropriate for either the individual level or the aggregate and institutional levels of analysis.

In this work, norms are viewed as having two major dimensions: a behavioral dimension and an expectation dimension. As Bierstedt (1970) has pointed out, a rule that is not followed by anyone is not a rule. Therefore, all rules must show up as patterns of behavior, or else they are not rules. The fact that we form expectations is probably more tied to the behavioral pattern than it is attributable to the moral "ought" or "should" often associated with norms. For example, in some cities the prevailing behavioral pattern when driving is to run yellow traffic lights; the expectation that people will engage in this behavioral pattern guides driving behavior. However, most people would be reluctant to say one "ought" to run yellow lights, even though this guides their own behavior and their expectations of others' behavior at an intersection.

The notion that norms are rules provides a key to the understanding of the basic concept. Max Black (1962) offers an illuminating discussion on the nature of rules. Black points out that a rule can have many different linguistic "formulations" and yet there is only one rule. For instance, the rule that one should parallel-park along a street can be formulated as "Park with the right side of the car close to and parallel to the curb" or "Park with the front and rear of the car at a 90° angle with the right-hand side of the street and the right side of the car close to the curb." Regardless of the number of equivalent formulations of a rule, the rule's meaning is that it forbids, permits, or requires an action for a class of actors in a situation. Thus, the rule regarding parallel parking requires a particular class of actors (automobile drivers) to act so as to park their vehicles parallel to the curb. Other examples of rules can be found in the formulation of games. For instance, it is the rule in chess that when a pawn (an actor) moves to the last rank on the board opposite its end, it may be exchanged for another piece. This example draws attention to the fact that a rule formulation relates the elements of an actor in a certain situation (position), an act, and the modality for that act (i.e., whether it is required, forbidden, or permitted).

A social norm is a rule regarding social behavior. Hence, *a social norm either permits, forbids, or requires a class of social actors (position) to act in a certain way*. For instance, the North American norm regarding adultery forbids adultery to both spouses. In previous times in South America, the norm regarding adultery was different for the husband (permitted) than for the wife (forbidden). By implication, if we were to accumulate all the rules for any one class of social actors (position) at a point in time, this accumulation of norms would represent the social role. Thus, the social role of "husband" in North America in 1985 would include the norms about adultery, economic support, division of household labor, and so on. It is important to note at this point that the definitions of rules and norms do *not* include sanctions as a necessary element. In fact, the definition of a norm is independent of whether or not sanctions are attached to the norm.

Norms (qua rules) have one dominant characteristic: All norms are "instructions for behavior." Black (1962) would only partially agree with this characterization. He identifies four kinds of rules: rules as "regulations," rules as "instructions," rules as "maxims," and rules as "principles." The four types of rules identified by Black can all be characterized as "instructions," and this clears up some of the complexity and confusion that his types engender. For instance, for Black a "principle" is a statement with a truth value. The very notion of a rule's expressing truth rather than convention is foreign to the social scientific meaning of norm. However, Black states:

> It is as if the speaker were to say "If you want to remember and distinguish the two kinds of cases that arise in electrostatic phenomena, bear in mind the formula 'Like poles repel, unlike attract.' " So construed, as mnemonic devices, rules in the principle-sense can be brought into not very distant relation with the instruction-senses of "rule" previously considered. (1962, pp. 113–114)

Thus, Black's formulation suggests that this most difficult of his types of rules (rules as principles with truth values) can be construed as a form of instruction.

The view that norms are rules instructing us to behave in a certain way seems consistent with the way in which norms are used in the social sciences. The most notable absence of "sanctions" in this characterization is a significant departure from the way in which Marini (1984) characterizes norms. In the sense used here, norms may or may not have sanctions of various strengths attached to them. Sanctions become one of two dimensions on which norms can be measured. Hence, any norm may vary from having no sanctions to having very strong sanctions attached to it. This view circumvents the problem that normative sanctions change over time though the norm (instruction) does not. There are even some norms with no sanctions attached that just function as maxims, such as "Transplant tomatoes outside after the last frost" and "A stitch in times saves nine." The important point here is that sanctions do not define all norms; they only define norms that function as regulations.

A second dimension on which norms can be measured is the qualitative dimension of which institution holds the norm and expresses the sanction if there is one. So, for example, many maxims originated in institutionalized religion but have lost the connection with other-worldly sanctions. Some norms are strongly sanctioned by several institutions; for example, the rules against homicide carry both religious and legal sanctions. Thus, the two measurement dimensions on which norms vary are the qualitative dimension of which institution (or institutions) holds the norm and the quantitative dimension of the strength of the sanctions attached to the norm.

Social scientists may identify norms in several ways. The most important factor in identifying a rule is the level of analysis on which the observation is conducted. If the individual level of analysis is used, then norms may be observed as the individual's morals. At the group level, norms may be observed as shared rules for behavior, such as "Hitting is not allowed in this family." At the aggregate level of analysis, the major way by which norms are identified is the observation of modal behavior. Another example from the game of chess illustrates these approaches. For instance, an individual might be asked why a certain move was made, and the response would be, "This is the *best* move [indicating the goal of winning the game] to be made in this situation." At the group level, the same question would be answered, "The move followed the constraints of the rules." There would be greater group consensus on the rules of the game than on the "best" move. At the aggregate level, the rules of the game could be inferred from the observation over time of many games. The rules would be those moves remaining invariant over time.

The fact that the constructs of social norms vary by the level of analysis is a point not often discussed by those with a primarily social-psychological (group-level) of reference. Scholars like Marini (1984) and Gibbs (1965) discuss norms as being defined primarily by social approval or disapproval. This is indeed an indicator of norms, but only for one level of analysis: It is restricted to regulatory group norms. Social approval or disapproval indicates those norms with some social group sanctions attached to them. Thus, observations using only approval–disapproval to indicate norms would miss norms with no sanctions, as well as norms that may only exist at some other level, such as the institutional level. Such observations would also miss norms that are interinstitutional, in the sense that the conjunction of a norm from one institution and that from another institution logically entails a norm that is in neither institution but is cross-institutional.

Black (1962, pp. 125–128) gives several examples illustrating how this situation arises. However, the most interesting example cited by Black is one in which he explores the possibility of inferring rules that are unformulated by the actors in a society. Imagine a society where all the rules are identified in a code book. However, the members of this society shy away from touching a fence; yet there is no taboo in the code book against the touching of the fence, nor will the inhabitants mention a taboo regarding the fence. As long as the behavior consistently appears to follow the rule that touching the fence is not allowed, the inference that there exists an unformulated rule is justified by the behavior pattern. Note that sanctions may not be observed when a norm is followed uniformly by all members of a society; however, this should not lead one to conclude that there is no rule governing this behavior. On the contrary, at the aggregate level, such an inference is justified.

The idea that there are interinstitutional or cross-institutional norms is especially important in relation to timing and sequencing norms. First, a simple example illustrates the logical way in which a norm in one institution may join with a norm in another institution to create a cross-institutional norm. Imagine a society in which the institutional family norm is that males should financially support their offspring. The educational institution in this society holds the rule that people must remain in school full-time until a certain age. The cross-institutional norm generated by the conjunction is that males should not have offspring until after a certain age. It may also be the case that if one asks people in this society whether there are rules governing the particular age at which a person should have offspring, they may say "No" until reminded of how the norms in other institutions conjoin with the family norms to create such rules.

The processes by which rules are developed are also different at each level of analysis. At the individual level, the individual learns rules as belonging to himself or herself. Thus, at the individual level, rules are primarily "internalized." This implies that at the individual level norms are seen by the individual as his or her own morals. At the group level of analysis, the group shares the rules through the process of "socialization." This process is characterized by social approval for the norms the group shares. At the institutional level of analysis, the process by which norms are developed is "institutionalization." This is the process whereby rules become either formal norms (codified) or behavior patterns. For example, many churchgoers receive the Eucharist with no understanding of its significance other than as ritual behavior.

The foregoing discussion is summarized in Table 9.1. Some clarification of this table is in order. For each level of analysis, there is a construct indicating the particular way of thinking about norms at each level. All of these constructs are part of the concept of norms as rules for social behavior, or, more precisely, rules that permit, forbid, or require an act for a class of social actors. Norms are instilled in individuals, groups, and institutions by very different processes. For instance, a rule for social behavior is learned and internalized by the individual so that

TABLE 9.1. Levels of Analysis for Norms

Level	Construct	Process	Sanctions
Individual	Morals	Internalization	Guilt
Group	Rules	Socialization	Approval
Institutional	Formal norms or behavior patterns	Institutionalization	Life chances

sanctions are internal (i.e., guilt and remorse). For each level, the sanctions are ones contained in the structure of the unit of analysis. So, the individual has the ability to feel strong emotions of guilt and remorse; the group has the ability to approve or disapprove; and the institution has the ability to deny or assist in life chances. "Life chances" include access to the opportunity structures in each institution, such as education, family, and work. What Table 9.1 is implying about the institutional level of analysis is that those people who do not follow the modal pattern of social behavior have differential access to institutional opportunities.

A concrete example may make this more clear. A male who drops out of high school is clearly not following the modal path in North America. Later in life, he will find that opportunities are denied him for this reason. Likewise, a male who completes a doctoral program is not following the modal pattern; he too will miss out on structural opportunities, such as delaying marriage and family or suffering family breakdown, as well as lost income. He may be starting his income earning and family when his contemporaries are sending their children off to college. He may be buying his first house years after others have acquired equity.

No one construct or level of analysis provides sufficient information for a truly valid inference of a social norm. The individual may feel guilt and remorse because of neuroses; the group may apply pressure for conformity as a test of loyalty, in addition to enforcing norms; and modal behavior may reflect systemic pressures other than normative ones. It seems, then, that a truly accurate inference of the existence and strength of a norm would necessitate measurement at all three levels of analysis. However, each construct taps a relatively independent dimension of social norms, which may be of interest in addressing particular research problems.

Some omissions from Table 9.1 demand attention. Notably, three levels of analysis that have been previously discussed are not included in the table. These are the relationship level, the aggregate level, and the interinstitutional level. The relationship level (which for present purposes includes any *n*-adic family subgroup) can be studied in exactly the same way in which groups are studied, since the dyad (or other subunit) is in fact a social group. The aggregate level is not directly included in Table 9.1 but is indirectly acknowledged. One way to infer institutional norms is to determine the modal behavior of the population in a social system. In this sense, the total aggregation or population is indicated by the institutional level of analysis. However, as previously discussed in Chapter 3, the aggregate level of analysis refers to subpopulations within the social system. For example, we may find that a population has a modal sequence of first job, first marriage, and first child. However, when we examine subsets of the population, such as ethnic aggregates or perhaps social class aggregates, we find that different modal paths exist among those subsets of the total aggregate or population. It is this level of analysis—subsets of the total aggregate or population—to which the aggregate level of analysis refers. The reason, then, why the aggregate level is not included in Table 9.1 is that inferences from the aggregate level are used to indicate a unique subset of the normative fabric of a society.

Much the same argument applies to the interinstitutional level. The inter- or cross-institutional level of analysis refers to those timing and sequencing norms that exist between social institutions. For instance, the norm indicating that young people should finish their education before getting married is a norm connecting the timing and sequencing of education with that of beginning a family. These cross-institutional norms can be researched with the same techniques used to research institutional norms.

The question of the validity of such inferences at the institutional and interinstitutional levels invariably arises. Clearly, there are historical periods when modal behavior does not reflect the normative content of institutions. For instance, behavior during episodes of war or pestilence, or the behavior of people *en masse,* may run counter to the content of institutionalized norms; the activity of a lynch mob is one example of counternormative mass behavior. In such cases, the modal behavior is not a valid indicator of the social norms. This problem is largely resolved by appropriate methodology. That is, institutional and interinstitutional social norms are indicated by relatively stable modal behavior over time. This is the principle of invariance under different conditions or treatments over time. Thus, the inference of interinstitutional or institutional norms from simple cross-sectional research must be viewed as having validity problems. The appropriate methodology would be either retrospective, cross-sectional/sequential, or longitudinal designs (see Chapter 5).

Marini's (1984) challenge to the normative model used in the study of development is based on an understanding of the concept of social norms that is appropriate to only one level of analysis. In fact, the concept of social norms as rules for social behavior is applicable to the individual, group, and institutional levels of analysis. From the population, inferences can be made regarding the institutional and cross-institutional levels. The idea of sanctions supplies a variable or dimension on which norms vary, rather than a necessary definitional component, as Marini suggests. A second dimension of norms is the qualitative variable of which institution (or institutions) hold the norm. Thus, Marini views norms as including only what I have defined here as the construct for norms with sanctions attached (regulatory norms) at the group level of analysis. Such a limited perspective on the concept of "norm" undoubtedly constricts and retards the analysis of family development. Marini's perspective would also deny the institutional aspect of norms and thus divert scholarly attention away from the higher orders of the social system. It seems doubtful that much understanding of family development can be gained unless there is an examination of the institutional and cross-institutional norms regarding the timing and sequencing of family stages.

HYPOTHESES

This section examines the hypotheses that the sequencing of different orders of cross-institutional events have effects on marital and work disruptions later in life, regardless of the marriage cohort. More precisely, it is hypothesized that fewer marital and work disruptions are associated with modal career patterns than with nonmodal career patterns. Gender is hypothesized to have a strong effect on sequencing, since the norms for males and females are quite different in most social institutions. Marital cohort is also hypothesized to have an effect on sequencing norms, since social-institutional norms change over time.

The set of events examined consists of first job, first marriage, and first child. The various orderings for these three events are hypothesized to have effects on later marital and work disruptions. More precisely, the modal orderings for males and females are hypothesized to have the lowest incidence of disruptions, because the modal orderings indicate the people whose lives are proceeding in accordance with both the institutional and the cross-institutional structure. The events included in this analysis are from two distinct institutions, work and family, as are the dependent variables of work and marital disruptions. It is expected that male and female orderings are different, since the institutional norms are gender-specific.

METHODS

Measures

The concept of "cohort" as discussed by Ryder (1965) may be applied to birth, marriage, or any other collectively shared characteristic. The particular problem faced by researchers analyzing the life span is the confounding of different effects that are all related to time (see Chapter 5). That is, the maturation of the individual, the effects of the historical period, and the birth cohort are interrelated. Each of these variables captures some important variance; however, the problems of multicollinearity and confounding are especially difficult ones in regard to them. Glenn (1977) and Morgan and Rindfuss (1985) discuss this problem. Morgan and Rindfuss (1985) conclude that only one of these variables can be included in a given analysis. In the present study, marriage cohort is used.

Marriage cohort appears to be the most valid way to capture the changing normative content of marriage. For example, it was almost a cliché of the 1970s that couples write their own wedding ceremonies. This practice, however, seems to have gone out of favor among those getting married in the 1980s and 1990s. A more serious change that would be captured by the marriage cohort is the difference between the definitions of marriage roles in the 1950s and the more equalitarian definitions of these roles in the 1970s. Undoubtedly, marriages change over time, and their nature is probably not determined completely by the prevalent institutional norms about marriage at the time of the marriage. However, it seems reasonable that the normative content specific to those marrying at certain periods may be better measured by marriage cohort than by either age at marriage or length of marriage. Thus, the choice here is to focus the analysis on the cohort effect rather than on maturation (age) or historical period.

Gender-specific norms are found in every social institution. The institutional norms governing work and family must take into consideration the gender of the person. It is especially obvious that gender is an area where cross-institutional norms have some considerable force. For example, the fact that females get pregnant and bear young during a reasonably specific time period in their life course must be taken into consideration in the norms governing work. The degree of correspondence between work career and family career for females has not been considered by researchers using the sequential approach. Morgan and Rindfuss (1985) investigated the effect of various sequences of the events of marriage, conception, and birth on women's marital disruption. Hogan (1978) examined the sequencing of the events of first job, completion of school, and marriage, and their effect on marital disruptions for males. However, there is no work comparing the differences in the ways males and females sequence the same events, and whatever differential effects these might have on marital disruption.

The major way to measure life event sequences is that developed by Hogan (1978), the Temporal Ordering Scale (TOS). This scale simply produces different categories for sequences. For example, as noted above, sequences in Hogan's work involved three events: first job, completion of school, and first marriage. Some of the various orderings were school–job–marriage and school–marriage–job. Morgan and Rindfuss (1985) used the same technique in their investigation, using the events of marriage, conception, and birth. The TOS is a categorical approach and constrains data analysis to frequency-based approaches such as log-linear analyses.

The events used in this study to form the TOS are a respondent's first job, first marriage, and birth of the first child. This set of events includes events from the two institutions of work and family, and indicates cross-institutional sequences. Events are considered simultaneous if they occurred in the same year (=). Events are considered serially ordered if they occurred in different years (-). The first sequence has 10 levels composed of the following orderings:

Job–marriage–child (J-M-C)
Job–child–marriage (J-C-M)
Marriage–job–child (M-J-C)
Marriage–child–job (M-C-J)
Child–job–marriage (C-J-M)
Child–marriage–job (C-M-J)
Child–job and marriage (C-J=M)
Job–marriage and child (J-M=C)
Marriage–child and job (M-C=J)
Job, marriage, and child simultaneously (J=M=C)

The second approach to the measurement of life event sequences is one I have developed (White, 1987a)—a scaling technique called the Career Conformity Scale (CCS). This technique is based on the theoretical rationale that a scale should measure the degree of conformity to the modal sequence for the life events under investigation. For instance, Hogan (1978) found that the modal sequence in his sample was school–job–marriage. The CCS, however, is computed as the extent of conformity to the mode for each time slot. So, for example, in the first time slot, the modal category for Hogan would be completion of school, and the mode for the second time slot would be first job. The scoring for the scale is computed by treating the frequencies for each event as a score. Thus, if 79% of the sample conformed to completion of school in the first time slot, then any individual would get a score of 79 for having that event in the first time slot, and any other event occurring for an individual at that time would be scored as its percentage frequency of occurrence for that time slot. As represented in Figure 9.1, an individual for whom these events occurred in the order school–job–marriage would get a high score. However, if one event was out of sequence, then at least two events would be nonmodal. This is a problem for both the CCS and the TOS. However, with the CCS, if the events are not modal but are nonetheless not far from the mode (in that they are relatively frequent events in those time slots), then the CCS score will still be high, since it is based on actual frequencies rather than simply the mode (as with the TOS). The CCS is thus a more accurate representation of the magnitude of conformity or deviance in the career sequence. I have provided a more detailed discussion elsewhere (White, 1987a).

Hogan (1978) and Morgan and Rindfuss (1985) both use marital disruptions as a dependent measure in their studies. Hogan's argument is that when one is not in synchrony with the normative sequencing of events, the effects of this dysynchrony may show up in various institutional areas. Since being out of step in one area has effects in other areas, it is difficult to identify the area in which consequences will appear. Marital disruptions are not unlikely, however, because the events normatively regulated in work and education have direct consequences for role performance and expectations in marriage. Morgan and Rindfuss (1985) examine events characteristic of the family and use marital disruptions as the dependent variable. Their use of marital disruptions as a dependent variable is entirely consistent with the events they use. Marital disruption (or stability) is used as a dependent variable in the present study because of the reasons cited by Hogan; it is also used in order to replicate the findings of previous studies. "Marital instability" refers here to whether or not the respondent was still living with his or her first spouse at the time of the survey.

The problem with the dependent variable of marital instability is that it only measures consequences in one institutional domain, the family. The second dependent variable used in this study is the number of work interruptions of at least 1 year's duration since the respondent first started working. This variable is chosen because it is a broad one

	Slot 1	Slot 2	Slot 3	
Possible events	Job Marriage School	Job Marriage School	Job Marriage School	
Sample % for event in modal time slot	School 79	Job 68	Marriage 75	Individual CCS score = 74 ([79 + 68 + 75]/3 = 74)

FIGURE 9.1. Example of Career Conformity Scale (CCS) scoring.

that is probably related to a multiplicity of causes, such as the number of children at home for the female and the degree of stress or stress-related illnesses for the male (e.g., alcoholism). Although this variable is inherently difficult to interpret, it is useful in spreading a wide net for possible effects in the work domain.

Data

The data for this study come from the 1984 Family History Survey. This data set, containing 14,004 cases, is discussed in some detail in Chapter 6. The selection of a subsample of those respondents who had completed all three events is necessary in order to examine the effects of various sequences of events. However, such a sample is limiting in several ways. The sample cannot be considered representative of the larger sample from which it is selected, and certainly not representative of the general population. Since only those who had completed these events at the time of the survey are included in the sample, there is the suspicion that certain age cohorts are severely misrepresented because of the problem of "right-censoring" (Tuma & Hannan, 1984). That is, people completing events in the most recent cohort would be more likely to have experienced premarital births and early marriages. The right-censoring of data also makes generalizations about marital disruptions and work interruptions very tenuous, since the time spent at risk would be longer for earlier cohorts than for more recent cohorts. There is no solution to such censoring problems, except to be cautious when examining the results, especially for the most recent cohort.

RESULTS

The portion of the sample completing all three of the life events—first job, marriage, and first child—is composed of 3,729 males and 3,631 females. The marital disruption for the event sample is given by the odds of staying married: an odds ratio of 4.88 to 1. This is a similar ratio to that for the larger sample of ever-marrieds (n = 10,472), which is 4.63 to 1. The gender-specific odds for staying married for ever-marrieds are 6.09 for males and 3.79 for females. This clear gender effect also shows up in the event sample, with odds for males' staying married of 6.41 and for females' staying married of 3.88. (This gender difference can in part be explained by the earlier age at marriage for females.) There is a slight difference in the age structure of the two samples, in that the larger sample (n = 14,004) shows odds of being female varying from 1.01 for those 18–25 years of age to a maximum difference of 1.18 for those 56–65 years of age. In the event sample (n = 7,614), the chance of being female for those 18–25 is 1.47, but this reverses to 0.95 for those 56–65 years of age. This indicates that those selected for the event sample are clearly different from the larger sample, in that there are more males in the older age groups than there are females. In earlier birth cohorts, it was often the case that women would never have worked, and so would not have completed all three events used for the selection of the event sample.

Those in the event sample had more work interruptions than those in the larger sample. For example, only 53.2% of the event sample reported no work interruptions of 1 year or longer, whereas 64.9% of the larger sample reported no work interruptions. The large percentage difference reflects the fact that the event sample must be older in order to have completed all three life events. The fact that the event sample is older accounts for the greater number of work interruptions in the sample, since these respondents would have had more work years at risk than the younger, larger sample.

The first hypothesis is that gender affects the way in which people sequence their life events. One way of documenting this gender difference is to examine the frequencies for various levels of the TOS for males and females (Table 9.2). For males, the three most frequent career sequences (TOS) are job–marriage–child (J-M-C), job followed by marriage and child in the same year (J-M=C), and job–child–marriage (J-C-M). For females, the three most frequent career sequences (TOS) are J-M-C, marriage–child–job (M-C-J), and J-M=C. The CCS also shows a gender difference, but the CCS appears to tap a different dimension from that measured by the TOS. In Table 9.2, for example, the CCS scores for both genders show different rank orderings than do those for the frequencies of the TOS. The rank orderings of CCS scores also differ for males and females, but do not match those for the TOS. There is a significant gender difference for both scales. The CCS scores suggest that for females, even though the sequences of J-C-M and marriage–job–child (M-J-C) are not as frequent as other sequences, they nonetheless conform to a normative structure. That is, the CCS scores for these sequences indicate that at least some of the events contained in the sequences are experienced in the same ordinal position as experienced by most others. The CCS scores for these two sequences thus suggest that some females in these categories were perhaps following a normative path, but were led to at least one event that was out of the normative sequence. For example, the sequence of J-C-M leads to the suspicion that these women were following the normative path (J-M-C), but that an unexpected pregnancy changed the order.

TABLE 9.2 Career Conformity Scale (CCS) Scores for Males and Females by Levels of the Temporal Ordering Scale (TOS)

	CCS					
TOS level	% males	*n*	Freq. rank	% females	*n*	Freq. rank
J-M-C	79.17	(2,790)	1	70.97	(2,430)	1
J-C-M	35.07	(209)	3	33.13	(118)	5
M-J-C	29.43	(107)	5	31.30	(138)	4
M-C-J	7.53	(159)	4	18.13	(651)	2
C-J-M	4.67	(61)	6	4.47	(59)	7
C-M-J	26.87	(20)	8	29.68	(68)	6
C-J=M	1.03	(12)	9	1.43	(14)	9
J-M=C	35.90	(363)	2	30.23	(264)	3
M-C=J	3.83	(59)	7	7.10	(33)	8
J=M=C	0.87	(32)	10	0.70	(27)	10

The second hypothesis is that people of different marriage cohorts sequence their life events in different ways. Table 9.3 shows that there are distinct differences among cohorts in the sequencing of early life events, even though all cohorts share the same sequence (J-M-C) as the modal sequence. For example, the most frequent sequence (J-M-C) is at an all-time low for males and females married in the 1980s. The decades of the 1950s through the 1970s appear to have greater conformity to the modal category of J-M-C than the marriage cohort of the 1980s. (The exception to this is the cohort married before 1940; however, the frequencies for this cohort are too small to be considered stable.) An additional caution must be added in comparisons using the 1980–1984 cohort. As previously discussed, this most recent cohort contains only those completing all three events. Clearly, this means that this sample cohort is not representative of those who got married during this time, and that the people in this sample cohort had not had the same amount of time at risk for marital disruption and work interruptions as earlier marriage cohorts.

Gender effects remain within the marriage cohorts. Those married in the 1940s offer a good example of such a gender difference. Although males in this cohort tended to conform to the modal pattern of J-M-C, almost 30% of the females experienced the sequence M-C-J. By contrast, in the marriage cohort of the 1970s, the sequence of M-C-J is not very frequent among females (5.9%). Table 9.3 thus demonstrates that the sequencing of these three life events has changed in part according to the

TABLE 9.3. Sequence of Life Events (TOS) by Marriage Cohort and Gender

Marriage Cohort	J-M-C	J-C-M	M-J-C	M-C-J	C-J-M	C-M-J	C-J=M	J-M=C	M-C=J	J=M=C	Total
1939 and before											
M	5		2	3	1				1	1	13
	(38.5)		(15.4)	(23.1)	(7.7)				(7.7)	(7.7)	(29.5)
F	9			20				2			31
	(29.0)			(64.5)				(6.5)			(70.5)
1940s											
M	310	8	14	39	3	4	1	25	16	1	421
	(73.6)	(1.9)	(3.3)	(9.3)	(0.7)	(1.0)	(0.2)	(5.9)	(3.8)	(0.2)	(45.2)
F	300	7	12	151	4	7		26	3	1	511
	(58.7)	(1.4)	(2.3)	(29.5)	(0.8)	(1.4)		(5.1)	(0.6)	(0.2)	(54.8)
1950s											
M	647	26	17	40	7	5	1	76	7	3	829
	(78.0)	(3.1)	(2.1)	(4.8)	(0.8)	(0.6)	(0.1)	(9.2)	(0.8)	(0.4)	(49.7)
F	553	21	15	171	8	16		50	4	5	843
	(65.6)	(2.5)	(1.8)	(20.3)	(0.9)	(1.9)		(5.9)	(0.5)	(0.6)	(50.4)
1960s											
M	760	58	19	50	12	4	4	129	12	15	1,063
	(71.5)	(5.5)	(1.8)	(4.7)	(1.1)	(0.4)	(0.4)	(12.1)	(1.1)	(1.4)	(52.1)
F	637	24	42	141	10	15	4	89	6	10	978
	(65.1)	(2.5)	(4.3)	(14.4)	(1.0)	(1.5)	(0.4)	(9.1)	(0.6)	(1.0)	(47.8)
1970s											
M	863	79	47	21	20	6	5	99	20	11	1,171
	(73.7)	(6.7)	(4.0)	(1.8)	(1.7)	(0.5)	(0.4)	(8.5)	(1.7)	(0.9)	(52.2)
F	766	47	56	63	22	17	7	71	18	7	1,074
	(71.3)	(4.4)	(5.2)	(5.9)	(2.0)	(1.6)	(0.7)	(6.6)	(1.7)	(0.7)	(47.8)
1980–1984											
M	138	38			18		1	33	3	1	232
	(59.5)	(16.4)			(7.8)		(0.4)	(14.2)	(1.3)	(0.4)	(54.5)
F	124	19	2	1	15	1	2	24	2	4	194
	(63.9)	(9.8)	(1.0)	(0.5)	(7.7)	(0.5)	(1.0)	(12.4)	(1.0)	(2.1)	(45.5)

Note. Each cell contains the percentage (in parentheses) of the specific gender and marriage cohort row total. The Total column contains the gender and marriage total *n*'s and in parentheses the percentage of the total for the specific marriage cohort. Grand totals and percentages: males, 3,729 (50.7%); and females, 3,631 (49.3%).

marriage cohort. It is also clear that the gender differences are getting smaller. There is a convergence toward the J-M-C modal sequence.

The third hypothesis is that the sequencing of early adult life events has an effect on later marital disruptions, independent of the effects of marriage cohort and gender. The present study approaches this problem in two ways. The TOS measures the frequency of each sequencing category (e.g., J-M-C). The CCS measures deviations from the modal category for each time point and is thus a quasi-metric. The TOS is analyzed first, using logit models.

The levels of the TOS, gender, and marriage cohort are each collapsed into only two levels or values, since with interaction terms problems with empty cells arise. The coding for the initial analysis is shown in Table 9.4. Since about 500 respondents did not complete all three events before a marital disruption, there are only 7,110 cases in this particular analysis. In many of the excluded cases, the person did not begin a first job until after a marital disruption. The exclusion of such cases is necessary if these events are to be treated as independent.

Table 9.5 shows the frequencies and odds for each level of the three independent variables. Clearly, the overall odds for the J-M-C category are much better than the odds for all other sequence categories. At every level of comparison, the J-M-C group has a better ratio for staying married. For example, males marrying before 1965 have an odds ratio of 7.68 still married for 1 no longer with his first spouse, compared to an odds ratio of 5.65 to 1 for all other sequences of the same gender and marriage cohort. Males marrying since 1965 have the best odds for staying married (15.58). It is somewhat misleading to compare the odds between marriage cohorts, because the marriage cohort also measures the length of time at risk in the marriage. Hence, it is probably not the case that more recent marriage cohorts will experience any less marital disruption than earlier cohorts when the time at risk is equal. This is, however, not the point of primary interest. The focus here is on showing that marriage cohort and gender affect the sequencing of events and that the sequencing of events affects marital disruptions. Table 9.5 shows that

TABLE 9.4. Coding for Variables in Log-Linear Analysis

Marital disruption	Event sequence	Marriage cohort	Gender
1 = Still married	1 = All others	1 = Before 1965	1 = Male
2 = Separated/ divorced	2 = J-M-C	2 = 1965 and after	2 = Female

TABLE 9.5. Frequencies and Odds for Sequence, Gender, and Marriage Cohort

			Independent variables			
Sequence	Gender	Cohort	% still married[a]	% sep./div.[a]	n^b	Odds
All others	M	Before 1965	84.9 (350)	15.1 (62)	412	5.64
		1965 and after	87.6 (502)	23.4 (71)	573	7.07
	F	Before 1965	85.9 (508)	14.0 (83)	591	6.12
		1965 and after	81.8 (463)	18.2 (103)	566	4.49
J-M-C	M	Before 1965	88.5 (1,122)	11.5 (146)	1,268	7.68
		1965 and after	93.9 (1,324)	6.0 (85)	1,409	15.57
	F	Before 1965	87.3 (931)	12.7 (136)	1,067	6.84
		1965 and after	91.6 (1,121)	8.4 (103)	1,224	10.88

[a]*n*'s are given in parentheses.
[b]Total $n = 7{,}110$

regardless of gender or marriage cohort, the modal sequence of J-M-C has a positive effect on staying married.

The saturated logit model yields five significant ($z = 1.96$) variables. All three main effects are significant, as are two two-way interactions. These five variables and their respective beta coefficients (Goodman, 1972) are presented in Table 9.6. These coefficients confirm the same relationships observed in the odds ratios in Table 9.5. The maximum-likelihood chi-square (L^2) indicates that this particular unsaturated model is a reasonable fit with the observed frequencies ($p = .620$). The negative coefficient for the main effect of sequence on marital disruption indicates that non-normative sequences are more likely to be associated with later marital disruption. As noted previously, females in this sample are more likely to have experienced a disruption in their first marriage than are males. Those married prior to 1965 are more likely to have experienced marital disruption than those married more recently, but this may simply be a result of the length of time at risk. Because the effect of marriage cohort may indicate the length of time at risk, it is unwise to interpret the two interactions containing marriage cohort. Perhaps the only point that should be discussed is that more recent cohorts in general seem to have had fewer disruptions in their marriages. In Canada, roughly 50% of all divorces occur within the first 13 years of marriage. Hence, those married up to 1965 would have been totally exposed to this risk period by 1978. The more recent marriage cohorts are still within this higher risk period for divorce and so may eventually show the same divorce rates. In the 1980s, however, there has been a slight decline in divorce rates, so we might expect that the more recent marriage cohorts may not

TABLE 9.6. Estimated Effects[a] of Sequence, Marriage Cohort, and Gender on the Likelihood of Marital Disruption

Variable	Coefficient	z
Sequence	−.26	−6.617
Gender	.114	2.948
Marriage cohort	−.132	−3.350
Sequence × marriage cohort	.161	4.074
Gender × marriage cohort	−.087	−2.280

[a]Unsaturated model, $L^2 = .957$, $df = 2$, $p = .620$.

reach the same levels of marital disruption as their predecessors. The present data indicate this trend but are not reliable indicators for the general population because of the selective nature of the sample.

A more detailed picture of the effect of the various sequences on marital disruption is afforded by a logit regression with all levels of the TOS. The analysis of the main-effects model shows that the five lowest estimates (intercepts) are for sequences in which the birth of the first child either preceded or was concurrent with the first marriage. This effect has been previously documented by Morgan and Rindfuss (1985). It seems that premarital births account in part for the relationship between the sequencing of these three events and marital disruptions. Most importantly, this finding leads to the concern that the effect found for sequencing is spurious and really based on the simple presence or absence of a premarital birth.

The question of spuriousness can be examined with the CCS. The CCS measures the deviations from the normative career sequence at each time point. A high score on the CCS represents conformity, and a low score represents deviance. Table 9.2 above shows the distribution of CCS scores by levels of the TOS. In order to further test the hypothesis regarding the way in which people sequence the early life events of first job, marriage, and child, a logit regression can be computed on the dependent binary variable of marital stability. The low score (0) on marital stability indicates that a respondent's original marriage was no longer intact at the time of the survey, and the high score (1) indicates that the respondent was still in the original marriage. Table 9.7 shows that premarital births have a negative effect on marital stability. The large ratio between the standard errors and the coefficients indicate that it is unlikely that these coefficients are 0. The negative effect for premarital births on marital disruption is roughly twice as great for females as for males. Marriage cohort appears to have a similar effect on marital stability for both genders. The CCS score has a small but not insignificant

TABLE 9.7. Logit Regression Coefficients for Premarital Births, Marriage Cohort, and CCS Score on Males' and Females' Marital Stability

	Regression coefficient	*SE*	Coeff./*SE*
Males			
Premarital birth	−.205	.095	−2.151*
Marriage cohort	.184	.023	8.001*
CCS score	.003	.001	2.567*
Females			
Premarital birth	−.437	.082	−5.307*
Marriage cohort	.184	.019	9.297*
CCS score	.003	.001	2.916*

*$p < .05$.

effect on marital stability. It is interesting to note that the CCS score is only slightly larger in effect (.004) when premarital births are excluded from the equation. This seems to indicate that premarital births have a significant effect on marital stability, independent of the CCS score. As suggested by the analysis of the TOS and marital disruption, this analysis of the CCS and marital stability indicates that premarital births have a significant effect but that sequencing continues to have a small but statistically significant effect when the effect of premarital births is controlled.

The normative sequencing of early life events may make it easier for people to coordinate their family careers with the sequences demanded by other institutions, such as work. In this study, the variable "number of work interruptions" is used to measure one possible outcome in the institution of work. This variable only includes work interruptions of at least 1 year in duration. Thus, it would seem reasonable that such prolonged absences from the labor force would have effects on such factors as seniority, promotions, and chances at career enhancement.

Table 9.8 presents an analysis of variance for the main effects of gender, marriage cohort, and event sequence on the number of work interruptions, while controlling for the number of children and whether or not the respondent left the labor force with the birth of the first child. These two control variables are added to the analysis because it is suspected that most work interruptions, especially for females, are accounted for by the fact that many mothers leave the labor force with the birth of the first child. Table 9.8 documents this effect, since the single largest contribution to explained variance is from the variable "left labor force with first child" ($SS = 2922.98$, $df = 1$, $p = .000$). With the covariates excluded from the equation, the main effects explain about

TABLE 9.8. Analysis of Variance for Number of Work Interruptions by Gender, Marriage Cohort, and Sequence with the Covariates of Leaving the Labor Force and Number of Children

	SS	*df*	*F*
Covariates			
Left labor force with first child	2,922.98	1	14,332.90*
Number of children	5.49	1	26.92*
Factors			
Gender	5.00	1	24.52*
Marriage cohort	16.37	5	16.05*
Sequence	22.16	9	12.07*
Explained	2,994.69	17	
Residual	1,497.29	7,342	
Total	4,491.98	7,359	
R^2 = .667			

*p = .000.

34% of the variance, as opposed to the 66% explained when the covariates are included. Although the three factors continue to have significant main effects, the size of these main effects is reduced considerably by the inclusion of the variable "left labor force with first child." This makes a most noticeable change in the sum of squares for gender (from 1,424.85 to 5.00 with the inclusion of the covariates). This suggests that women have a larger number of work interruptions, chiefly because they leave the labor force for child care. However, even after the effects of the covariates are removed, females still have a small but significant difference in work interruptions due to sequencing.

To examine the hypothesis concerning the effect of the conformity to the normative sequencing of events on the number of work interruptions, the CCS score is regressed (least squares) on the number of work interruptions. Table 9.9 and 9.10 show standardized regression coefficients for the CCS score on the number of work interruptions for females and males, respectively. In both tables, the beta for the CCS score represents the effect on the number of work interruptions, controlling for the number of children, leaving the labor force at the first birth, and marriage cohort. Clearly, conformity to the normative sequence of early life events has a significant effect on the number of work interruptions, over and above that of the other variables in the equation. For both males and females, the effect for career conformity is negative, indicating that those with the greatest conformity to the modal sequence experienced the fewest work interruptions.

TABLE 9.9. Regression for Number of Children, Leaving the Labor Force at the First Birth, Marriage Cohort, and CCS Score on the Number of Work Interruptions for Females (n = 3,063)

Variables (in order of entry)	R^2 change	Beta
Number of children	.009	–.009*
Left labor force at first birth	.426	.691**
Marriage cohort	.007	–.087**
CCS score	.006	–.087**

*p = .506.
**p = .000.

TABLE 9.10. Regression for the Number of Children, Leaving the Labor Force at the First Birth, Marriage Cohort, and CCS Score on the Number of Work Interruptions for Males (n = 3,728)

Variables (in order of entry)	R^2 change	Beta
Number of children	.004	.022*
Left labor force at first birth	.777	.880**
Marriage cohort	.002	–.054**
CCS score	.003	–.052**

*p = .009.
**p = .000.

DISCUSSION

The data strongly suggest that males and females tend to sequence the three life events examined here—first job, first marriage, and first child—in different ways. Although the modal category for the TOS (J-M-C) is the same for both genders, the rank orderings of all categories are quite different for males and females (Table 9.1). For example, the three most frequently occurring categories of the TOS for males were J-M-C, J-M=C, and J-C-M, whereas for females the ranking was J-M-C, M-C-J, and J-M=C. This may not seem such a large deviation, but it looks even more pronounced when one examines the gender difference for each marriage cohort in Table 9.3. For instance, in Table 9.3 it is clear that the greatest conformity to the modal career for males is in the marriage cohort of the 1950s. The greatest conformity to the modal career for females is in the marriage cohort of the 1970s. This difference in the percentages of these cohorts conforming to the modal career seems to suggest a shift over time in the gender norms governing cross-institutional sequencing of these events. These data suggest that the norms governing male event sequencing in the 1950s were unswervingly followed, as compared with the males in the 1970s marriage cohort. Certainly this finding goes along with the popular 1950s conception of the "organization man" and the "man in the grey flannel suit."

On the other hand, females during the 1950s appeared to enjoy considerably more freedom in sequencing these life events. That is, females did not demonstrate the same degree of conformity to one path until the marriage cohort of the 1970s. It is perhaps not surprising to many scholars that with all the pressure in the decade of the 1970s for women to work as well as have families, their early life event sequencing is as conformist as that for the males two decades previously. Overall, during the time covered by the marriage cohorts, females have tended to become less diversified and more conforming to the modal career pattern, whereas males have tended to become more diversified and less conforming to the modal career sequence since the marriage cohort of the 1950s.

Although the preceding discussion has concluded that there is an effect for marriage cohort on the sequencing of life events, it is impossible to distinguish whether this effect is a cohort, age, or period effect. All three are confounded in this analysis. For example, those married in the 1970s are from a relatively homogeneous age group that was exposed to the social and cultural influences of the 1970s, such as women's liberation. Glenn (1977) points out that these effects are confounded and that there exists no statistical means whereby these effects can be simultaneously separated.

In this study, marriage cohort has been used to measure the changes in social norms related to the sequencing of life events. Since age at marriage has shifted only slightly during the time covered in this study, it seems that it would not have a major effect. It appears more plausible that marriage cohort captures both cohort and period effects rather than age effects. The norms regulating the sequencing of life events undoubtedly interact with period events. For instance, the norms concerning working wives are responsive both to ideological movements such as women's liberation and to changes in legislation supporting affirmative action. There is a complex interaction between the events of a period and the normative structure of social institutions. The investigation of this interaction goes beyond the data available for the present study. However, it does seem reasonable to conclude that marriage cohort is related to the sequencing of life events, and that at least some of that relationship is due to changes in the institutional normative fabric.

As in previous studies (Hogan, 1978; Morgan & Rindfuss, 1985), non-normative sequences are associated with marital disruptions. The sequence of J-M-C appears to have significantly fewer marital disruptions than any other sequence, regardless of gender and marriage cohort. The analysis of the CCS (Table 9.7) indicates that the positive effect for conformity on marital stability is the same, regardless of gender and cohort. Though males and females have different degrees of variation in the sequencing of events, conformity to their gender-specific sequencing has a positive effect on staying married.

Sequencing also has a significant effect on work interruptions. For example, the analysis of the TOS in Table 9.8 shows that those respondents following the modal sequence of J-M-C had the fewest work interruptions. The analysis of the CCS suggests a similar conclusion. Tables 9.9 and 9.10 indicate that when the effects of the number of children and leaving the labor force at the birth of the first child are controlled, both males' and females' CCS scores are negatively related to the number of work interruptions. The large effect size for leaving the labor force at the birth of the first child identifies one of the main components in female work interruptions—that is, the birth and care of offspring. However, it is also important to note that for females there remains a significant effect for the CCS score, suggesting that sequencing remains an important dimension.

CONCLUSION

The norms that comprise our social institutions change slowly. Likewise, the cross-institutional norms governing the synchronization of various institutional expectations for individuals change slowly. For example, in the present study one sequence of three events—first job, first marriage, and first child—has been found consistently to be the modal category for all marriage cohorts from 1940 through 1984. This finding seems to document the relatively phlegmatic process of institutional change. However, this study has also found that the degree of conformity to this "normative" sequence varies by both gender and marriage cohort. In fact for males married in the decade of the 1950s there was the greatest conformity to this modal sequence. Females showed greater conformity to the modal sequence if they married in the decade of the 1970s. Since the events composing the sequence in this study are from two different institutional domains, it is plausible to conclude that although the cross-institutional norms do not appear to have changed, the degree of conformity to those norms does seem to have changed. This conformity to those norms about the sequencing of life events is itself a measure of the ways and means by which the normative structure within and between social institutions changes.

The process of change is not a painless one for the individuals involved. Since one initial step in institutional change is nonconformity or norm breaking by individuals, it is possible to conceptualize the dysynchrony of individuals' sequencing of events as a type of rule breaking. This norm breaking can be looked at as a necessary part of social change. However, sanctions are traditionally attached to the breaking of norms. The types of sanctions at the institutional level of analysis are different from those at the group level. What sanctions are applied to those who deviate from the cross-institutional norms about sequencing of events? Hogan (1978), for males, and Morgan and Rindfuss (1985), for females, have both reported significantly higher rates of marital disruption for those who do not follow the normative path for sequencing life events, even though they did not use the same events in their studies. In the present study, this finding regarding marital disruption is replicated for yet another cluster of event sequences. In addition, since the sequencing includes events from both work and family, this study has found that those following non-normative sequences have more work interruptions than those following the normative path. Work interruptions should be negatively related to career opportunities and seniority. As indicated in Table 9.1, lowered life chances are conceptualized as a "sanction" at the institutional level of analysis. Thus, it seems that the sanctions attached to non-normative sequencing of events are disruptions in both areas of work and family later in life.

There must be some positive benefits to such nonconformity in the sequencing of life events. If these events had no positive components but only negative sanctions, it would be doubtful that such sequences would be pursued except by accident or ignorance. The systematic deviations found in this study and other studies suggest the opposite. There are probably different historical reasons for the deviance, which this study has not attempted to measure as period effects. In addition, delaying marital and family responsibilities probably has benefits for particular occupations. For such groups, it will be interesting if in fact deviance in their career sequence, in addition to timing, continues to have negative effects on marital stability. It will be even more interesting if, for certain groups, the relationship between career deviance and marital stability is positive. These questions are only some of the many questions this study poses for future research.

Hogan (1978) explains the effects of dysynchrony as being out of step both between and within institutions. Once one is out of step in one institution, there are problems in meeting the expectations of other institutional domains as well. For example, a premarital pregnancy obviously affects the time available for the labor force, as well as the probability of continuing education.

The question that seems most acutely in need of further research is whether or not the effects reported for dysynchronous event sequences are not in fact due to one particular event, such as premarital pregnancy. It may be the case that what is being measured by the event sequences is simply one efficacious event. If this were found to be so, then attributing effects to the sequencing of events would be specious. However, there is some indication in this study that this is not the case (see Tables 9.8, 9.9, 9.10). For instance, when the event variables for leaving the labor force at the birth of the first child and the number of children are controlled for, the sequencing still has a significant effect on work interruptions. The question is not resolved by this one example; certainly there is a need to go further in analyzing the independent effects of events, their sequencing, and their timing on other criterion variables.

CHAPTER 10

Family Deviance and Change

In the preceding chapter, the crux of the argument is that cross-institutional norms appear to exist and to have effects on later life events. One important question arising from that analysis is this: "Is it the deviance itself that leads to these later life disruptions, or is it really an effect of certain event sequences?" This question asks whether deviance in one area of social life, such as in the sequencing of early life events, simply continues as an individual or family trait (as "trait" is used in personality psychology) in the sequencing of later life events. If this were true, then the effects found in Chapter 9 would be spuriously attributed to certain event orderings rather than to the general trait of deviance. These questions are difficult ones to address, since early event deviance is correlated with later event deviance. The question is whether this correlation is the result of the particular deviant early event sequences, or of a general trait of deviance expressed throughout the life span in certain individuals, dyads, and families.

This chapter addresses these questions in two ways. First, it attempts to clarify terminology and, in fact, the very notion of the relation between change and deviance. Second, an empirical analysis of two types of career deviance examines the effects for deviance in early cross-institutional events and events within the institution of the family. The hypothesis here is that if the effects for these two different patterns are the same, then the proposition that effects are due to some general pattern of deviance, resembling a family or individual trait, would appear as more plausible than the proposition that the events themselves make a difference. More precisely, if cross-institutional event deviance and within-institution deviance have similar effects, then one must conclude that the hypothesis regarding general deviance as a trait is more likely than the normative interpretation, since cross-institutional norms should have a different effect size from that of institutional norms.

Understanding why this is so requires a more detailed discussion of how cross-institutional and institutional norms work.

DEVIANCE AND TYPES OF CHANGE

The notion of "deviance" is inherently ambiguous (Datan, 1983). It includes the two meanings of (1) deviance as an infrequent form of behavior, and (2) deviance as norm breaking. As previously discussed in Chapter 9, the connection between these two meanings has been a subject of scholarly debate (Marini, 1984). The resolution of this debate lies in the view of norms as having two dimensions. One is that of the strength of any negative sanctions attached to the norm. This dimension of norms is especially useful at the individual, dyadic, and group levels.[1] A second dimension is that of the frequency of behavior or conformity to the norm. This is really a measure of the norm's existence in behavior at the institutional level. These two dimensions—behavioral frequency (institutional level) and approval–disapproval (group level)—are useful at different levels of analysis. It must, however, be clear that the necessary and sufficient condition for the inference of a norm is the frequency-of-behavior dimension and not the sanction dimension. Otherwise, we could be caught in the trap of maintaining rules as norms, even though no one follows these rules.

Whereas the idea of normative deviance is simply ambiguous because it contains two dimensions, the notion of "change" is more difficult because its everyday use is vague and amorphous. In Chapter 7, three types of change have been identified: "developmental change," "evolutionary change," and "random change." When one is discussing change, it is wise to identify which type of change one is considering. Each type is a different process with different meanings and types of outcomes. Certainly the general outcome of change is that things are not the same as they were. However, this is a ludicrous statement from a scientific perspective.

Not only is it necessary to be precise in identifying which type of change we discuss, but it is also important to focus on the level or levels of analysis at which we are discussing change. It is true that a change in one part of a social system is usually associated with changes in other parts, but such global thinking adds little to our understanding of change. For example, the statement "The family is undergoing change" has very different meanings, depending on which level of analysis is being considered and which type of change. At the group level, a family may change developmentally, and hence "change" refers to a transition from one state to another. The family may also change at the institutional level, but at this level we are referring to a change in the norms governing family life. This normative change may be part of the development of the institution or adaptation to changes in other institutions. These two different meanings of "family change" illustrate the importance of identifying both the level of analysis and the type of change in any such discussion.

The types of change need to be further elaborated. "Developmental change" is, by this time, the most familiar. Developmental change is a process in which the probability of a transition to a new state is dependent on both the present state and the duration of time in the present state. At the group or subgroup level, developmental change is characterized by the relatively systematic transition between stages of the family. The stages are defined by norms regulating the roles and role relationships within the family. The transitions are regulated by timing and sequencing norms. Thus, finally, development is explained by the institutional norms.

This is not to say that all family group change is explained by those institutional norms, since not all family change is developmental change. Clearly, the family group is always surrounded by other social institutions, which sometimes make contradictory demands on the group. In responding to these demands, a family may choose to deviate from one set of institutional norms in order to follow another set of institutional norms. Also, a family group is always part of a larger environment that includes other societies and processes. For instance, this larger environment includes processes such as urbanization and events such as war and depression, which are beyond any one society's institutional frame.

A second type of change is "evolutionary change." Evolutionary change is of two sorts. The more familiar of these to social scientists is natural selection. Natural selection is the process by which change in the norms of some institution (e.g., political or economic institutions) creates a disjunction with the norms of another institution (e.g., the family). The subsequent changes in response to this normative disjunction are perceived by social scientists as either "adaptive" or "maladaptive" on the basis of the realignment of cross-institutional norms. Thus, evolutionary change is commonly discussed under the rubric of "adaptation." The family as a group may adapt to the social norms of the institution, or the institution of the family may adapt to the norms of other institutions. In this sense, adaptation means articulation with the institutional norms, though not literally conformity to them.

A second sort of evolutionary change is change in genetic substance, usually called "mutation." In relation to social groups and institutions, this is a much more foreign concept than is adaptation or natural selection. This is because social science at this time lacks a well-developed genetic theory of the social system, even though we do have a relatively well-developed ecological theory of the social system (e.g., Bronfenbrenner, 1979; Featherman, 1985; Hannan & Freeman, 1977). Social mutations must be those forms of normative deviance that arise spontaneously in families and the institution of the family. As such, they are relatively unpredictable at this time and may as well be considered as a type of random change.

The last type of change is "random change." Random change is nonsystematic, in that either the probability of an occurrence is its base rate ($1/n$), or the occurrence is so rare (as in the case of mutations) as to have no computable probability.

This chapter is principally concerned with the two major forms of systematic change, developmental change and adaptive change. As we shall see, developmental changes take place mainly within institutions and groups, whereas cross-institutional changes must be analyzed as a form of adaptation.

CHANGE AND LEVELS OF ANALYSIS

The different types of change can be seen operating in different ways at each level of analysis. All of these changes take place in the global context of certain processes. For example, there is a global process of moving from agrarian-based economies to postindustrial economies. Another global process is the move from rural communities to urban settings. Yet another global process is the move from social values favoring group solidarity to those values favoring individual gratification. Determining which of these is cause and which is effect is beyond the scope of the current enterprise; however, it is important to note that all societies function within this context. It should also be kept in mind that these global processes are not sufficient to explain the changes within the groups and institutions of any particular society. Rather, it is more important for us to understand the different types of change and how they operate at different levels of analysis.

Group Level

At a group level such as the family, change may be either systematic or random. The immediate concern is with forms of systematic change in the family group. As seen in previous chapters, one form of family change is developmental. In developmental change, the norms constructing roles and role relationships shift from stage to stage.

Another form of change for the family group is adaptation to the norms of social institutions other than the institution of the family. The family institution changes slowly. Other social institutions may change their norms leaving the family's timing and sequencing norms in a state of disjunction with those of the other institutions. In this case, families may change their behavior in line with that of the other institutions in society, even though this behavior may deviate from the institutional norms of the family. This is actually a form of deviance when viewed from the perspective of the institution of the family, but it is also a form of adaptation (or conformity) when viewed from the perspective of other social institutions.

An example of this process is the shift toward cohabitation as a form of premarital mate selection. The family institutional norms have been slow in changing. However, the norms regarding women in the labor force and prolonged education make cohabitation a viable means for women to establish a relationship without undertaking the pressures to bear children, because the next step is marriage and after that step comes children. In addition, cohabitation allows both partners to finish their education and begin occupational careers before undertaking the potentially stressful transitions of marriage and childbirth. Thus, this behavior, which is viewed as deviant within the institution of the family, may be seen as corresponding well with the norm to get married after the completion of education and start of a job.

It is an important characteristic of this type of deviance that as the frequency of the norm breaking increases, the norms within the institution of the family change. This form of deviance within an institution but conformity to the norms of other institutions is a means by which an institution adapts its norms to, and coordinates them with, the norms of other institutions in a social system. It must be kept in mind, that the deviance–conformity here is on the group level. That is, individual families (or individuals, in the case of cohabitation) decide to break norms within one institution in order to conform to norms in another institution. The dominant characteristic of this type of evolutionary adaptation by groups, individuals, and dyads is that there are shifts at the aggregate level in the frequency of behavior (deviance) preceding shifts in sanctions at the group level (Modell, 1980).

Institutional Level

Most of the change that takes place in the norms of an institution comes about by means of the increasing frequency of deviance at the group level. However, there is some change at the institutional level that is developmental. That is, like groups, institutions undoubtedly have stages of development. This means that at some point deviance from institutional norms precipitates changes in the normative fabric, such that the preceding set of norms is qualitatively distinct from the emergent set not being followed in the social system. It is not possible at this time to identify the developmental stages of institutional change. Developmental change in institutions should in retrospect be perceived as a normal transition in the life span of the institution, such as increasing structural diversification. Hence, the division of the institution of kinship into the areas of marriage, family, and kinship is considered a relatively natural developmental change in the course of the institution.

One fact about institutions is clear: Their dominant characteristic is inertia. Institutions not only are slow to change, but are often resistant to change. Given this fact, it is nonetheless possible to speculate as to the nature of this slow and gradual change. Hannan and Freeman (1984) discuss the life cycle variations in inertia for large organizations. Some of the same characteristics may be found in institutions. For example, the inertia of institutions may increase monotonically with age. This also implies that there is a corresponding resistance to spontaneous forms of change. One of the most intriguing characteristics in this regard is suggested by Hannan and Freeman (1984) in their discussion of "organizational death rates":

> If the liability of newness reflects internal processes, the death rate will jump with structural changes. In contrast, if the decline in the death rate with age reflects mainly the operation of external processes of legitimacy and exchange, the death rate will not jump when structural changes do not imply a change in basic goals. That is, arguments about internal and external processes lead to different predictions about the effect of structural reorganization on the death rate. (p. 160)

What this passage implies about institutional change is that when change comes from within the institution, as in cases where group behavior is increasingly deviant from the norms of the institution, the institution may be more resistant to change. But when external institutions and environmental forces compel changes, there may be less institutional resistance to change. Thus, it would seem that external forces, at the same time as they require coordination of norms, demonstrate the legitimacy of the institution; by contrast, deviance from within threatens the goals and legitimacy of the institution. For instance, change from within the institution of the family may be met with greater resistance than changes that the institution of the family needs to make in order to adapt to the timing and sequencing of events in educational and work careers.

Evolutionary change in the institution comes about principally by means of adaptation. Norms in one institution are adjusted into line with norms in other institutions. This is adaptive change as long as the changes are extensions of the basic goals of the institution. This type of change should not be confused with developmental change, since it may not necessarily involve a transition to a different state. Rather, adaptive change is an adjustment to the normative content of other institutions. For example, the norm requiring increased competence in the labor force, and hence increasing the intrusions by educational organizations into family socialization, is viewed as an adaptive change rather than as a developmental change of state for the institution of the family.

Cross-Institutional Level

The timing and sequencing norms that coordinate the various institutional normative structures in a social system develop and evolve over time. Developmental change in the cross-institutional norms is difficult to imagine, since it would entail a sweeping view of social development. Such a perspective would involve the identification of configurations of institutional norms with cross-institutional norms that would represent distinct stages of social development. This represents a mammoth scholarly undertaking, and as yet remains a remote theoretical possibility.

It is a much more manageable task to identify the process of adaptation (evolutionary change) in cross-institutional norms. Cross-institutional norms change in response to individuals' or families' inability to follow the norms of several different social institutions. This incapacity is usually caused by a normative demand overload on individuals or families. For example, people may begin showing the effects of high stress loads because several different institutions require simultaneous developmental transitions within each institution (Hill & Mederer, 1983; Pearlin, 1980).

Another form of adaptive change in cross-institutional norms is that seen in response to external social forces such as pestilence. Changes in the norms that synchronize the timing and sequencing of events in institutions such as education, politics, religion, the economy, and the family are even more resistant to change than institutional norms, since these cross-institutional norms link these institutions with one another and insure a more or less functional social system. The external forces that may compel change must be sufficient in duration to create cross-institutional adaptation. For example, there seem to be few adaptations of cross-institutional norms to relatively short-lived events such as war or depression (e.g., Elder, 1974). On the other hand, a long-lived event such as the plagues of the Middle Ages might be expected to create changes in cross-institutional timing and sequencing norms. The event that creates the impetus for change may be a random event, but the response of adaptation is clearly a form of systematic change. Historical research must identify the duration and types of world events that are responsible for adaptive changes in cross-institutional norms. After all, these norms are close to the very essence of any social system.

INSTITUTIONAL AND CROSS-INSTITUTIONAL DEVIANCE

There is a significant difference between institutional deviance and cross-institutional deviance. Institutional deviance is an individual's or group's failure to conform to the norms within one institution (e.g., the family). As previously mentioned, this form of deviance is most often motivated by conformity to norms in other institutions that do not coordinate well with the norms in the other institution. For example, educational norms are increasingly formalized to provide educational organizations with access to children at earlier and earlier ages. On the other hand, family norms emphasize increasing amounts of time for parental forms of nurturance. Work norms emphasize increasing degrees of commitment and time for people in the labor force, including mothers, to work. Clearly, these diverse demands come at approximately the same age and stage of the family. The result is bound to be that if the family members conform to one set of institutional norms, they violate a set in some other institution. This is a relatively clear-cut case in which some form of institutional deviance will result. When one behavioral response (institutional deviance) becomes a frequent violation of the norms within an institution, those norms will gradually shift to favor the behavior. Thus, placing infants and toddlers in day care in the 1950s was considered quite deviant. In the 1980s and 1990s, day care for very young children, though not the norm, has become so frequent as to be tolerated (if not favored) in North America. Undoubtedly, if the work and educational norms do shift, then day care and the norms about family nurturance of the young will change. This example also provides an illustration of the resistance to normative shifts resulting from this type of deviance, because day care was for a while considered a threat to the very institution of the family. Such beliefs are likely to emerge whenever deviance occurs at the individual or group level and involves the violation of a norm within an institution (institutional deviance).

The case of cross-institutional deviance is quite different. Cross-institutional deviance is failure to conform to the timing and sequencing norms between or among institutions. In other words, this form of deviance always involves at least two institutional domains. For example, if cross-institutional norms favor people's first completing their education, then starting their first jobs, and thereafter getting married, any shift in this sequence involves at least two institutional areas. However, it is important to keep in mind that the norms within those institutions may not be violated; the norms being violated are the cross-institutional norms. For example, a medical student who marries before completing the educational program and before starting a job may nonetheless follow the sequencing norms within the family. The norms that are violated are the prevailing sequencing and timing norms, which are cross-institutional and not institutional. This is not to say that cross-institutional deviance may not be associated with institutional deviance, but that there is no necessary connection. The two forms of deviance can operate independently.

HYPOTHESES

The primary hypothesis of the present study is that deviance in career sequencing is associated with an increased probability of disruptions later in life. Although this point has been considered in Chapter 9 by means of the Temporal Ordering Scale (TOS), part of that analysis is reconsidered in this chapter with a more direct measure of deviance, the Career Conformity Scale (CCS). This approach allows a more direct interpretation of deviance than does the other approach.

Institutional deviance and cross-institutional deviance can be independent of each other. For example, a pattern of cross-institutional deviance such as getting married prior to completing one's education and beginning one's first job may not be related to following the normative pattern of events within an institution, such as marriage preceding the birth of the first child. One can easily get married before completing education and first job, and still not have an out-of-wedlock birth. Thus, a second hypothesis is that cross-institutional deviance and institutional deviance have independent effects.

If cross-institutional deviance and institutional deviance are related, then there are two plausible hypotheses, either of which might account for such a relationship. One hypothesis is that the cross-institutional and institutional norms are linked in some way, so that a deviant pattern in one area facilitates or determines deviance in the other area. So, for example, out-of-wedlock births are more probable among young people still in school. The institutional family norm regarding out-of-wedlock births is for the young parents to get married. This event of marriage, however, will then result in a deviant pattern from the cross-institutional sequencing norms, which favor the sequence (1) completion of education, (2) first job, and (3) marriage (Hogan, 1978). However, such dependences as given in this example should not be the case for later age groups. Thus, this hypothesis can be further clarified by controlling for age at marriage.

The second hypothesis that might explain a relationship between institutional and cross-institutional deviance is that some individuals, dyads, or families have a predilection toward normative deviance, which is expressed in both the domains of institutional norms and cross-institutional norms. This perspective argues that deviance is similar to a trait and that it is expressed in several areas. One problem with this trait argument is that in order to explain increases and decreases in deviance, explanations must appeal to changes in the distribution of a trait rather than changes in the social context. For example, if individuals are deviant because of an inherent trait, then increases in deviance must mean that there are more of that type of individual. This is clearly a more social-genetic theory than a social-ecological theory. Nonetheless, this is an alternative hypothesis when institutional and cross-institutional deviance are strongly related.

METHODS

The most general hypothesis in regard to career deviance is that those traversing a more deviant career pattern early in life show greater marital instability later in life. This point has been discussed and documented in Chapter 9, using a categorical approach developed by Hogan (1978), the TOS. In the present analysis, this point is repeated with another approach that more closely measures deviance, the CCS.

The CCS (White, 1987a) is a more adequate measure for some forms of deviance. It is designed to measure the degree to which an individual's career sequence of events deviates from the modal ordering of events. The CCS has two alternative ways of approaching this problem. First, a modal career (e.g., job–marriage–child) can be identified, and the deviations of other career orderings for these events can be computed on the basis of the frequency of occurrence. The more frequent patterns are closer to the mode and hence less deviant. This approach has the drawback that one infrequent event in a career sequence (e.g., a spouse's death) can produce a high deviance score, even though all the other events conform to the modal pattern. To get around this problem, a second method of computing the CCS can be used. This second approach computes a deviance score for each position in an event sequence. For example, the event sequence job–marriage–child has three event positions. In the first event position, the most frequently occurring event is the first job. Any individual obtaining a first job in this position is given the frequency percentage for that event. Thus, if 79% of the sample has a job as the first event, that would be the score for each individual who has that event in the first position. In the second position, the most frequent event is marriage. Someone who begins a job in the second position would receive the CCS score based on the percentage frequencies for that second position. Clearly, having a job as the first event results in a high score, whereas having a job as the second event results in a lower score, since marriage is the modal event in the second position. This second approach to the computation of the CCS maintains independence between event scores, so that one deviant event does not misrepresent an otherwise nondeviant career sequence. This second approach to the computation of the CCS is the one used in this study. (Readers may refer to the previous discussion in Chapter 9 for additional detail on the computation of the CCS.)

The events used here to construct the CCS are first job, first marriage, and first child. These are the same events used in Chapter 9, so that comparisons with the analysis in that chapter are facilitated. The CCS is constructed from the frequencies for events for each ordinal position (or time slot) in the sequence. So, for example, the sequence of job–marriage–child contains three ordinal positions. For each ordinal position, the percentage of the frequencies for the three events are treated as scores. Thus, in the first ordinal position for males, the event scores are as follows: job = 763, marriage = 195, child = 35, and all three events occurring simultaneously = 7. Each of these scores represents the percentage occurrence to one decimal place (e.g., 763 = 76.3%). A high score on the CCS represents greater conformity to the modal pattern of sequencing events. Although one deviant event may still pull the CCS score down, it has much less effect than when the entire sequence is scored by its percentage frequency. Separate CCS scores are computed for males and females, since the two genders have different frequencies for these events. The reliability for these two scales appears fairly high. Elsewhere (White, 1987a), I have reported a Cronbach's alpha for the male CCS as .857 and for the female CCS as .887.

In order to examine the relationship between cross-institutional and institutional deviance, the three events used in the CCS must be partitioned into institutional and cross-institutional orderings. The TOS developed by Hogan (1978) is a very useful means for comparing cross-institutional and institutional deviance, since it allows examination of the event orderings. The cross-institutional sequence examined in this chapter is the event ordering of first job and first marriage. This sequence contains an event from each of the two institutions of work and family. Within the institution of the family, the events examined are first marriage and first child. Thus, it is entirely possible that deviance in the cross-institutional sequence (here, marriage preceding first job) is not related to any corresponding deviance in the sequencing of marriage and first child.

The dependent variable in this analysis is staying married. "Staying married" refers to a respondent's still being with his or her first spouse at the time of the study; it does not refer to remarriage or common-law unions. Those no longer married include respondents in the categories of separated, divorced, and "other," but not those who were no longer married because of the death of a spouse.

RESULTS

The data used for this analysis are derived from the same subset of cases from the Family History Survey used in Chapter 9. The results are presented in two sections. First, the two simple patterns for institutional and cross-institutional events are analyzed separately. After that, the second section examines the total effect for a deviant career composed of all three events and uses the CCS to measure deviance.

Institutional and Cross-Institutional Sequences

In Chapter 9, a distinct gender difference has been found to exist for the sequencing of events. That is to say, there appear to be distinct norms for males and females. In the present analysis, results are presented for each gender. Table 10.1 presents the percentages for males staying married, partitioned by cross-institutional and institutional sequences; Table 10.2 presents similar data for females.

A comparison of Tables 10.1 and 10.2 shows a gender difference similar to the one found in Chapter 9. In regard to the cross-institutional sequencing of first job and first marriage, it is interesting to note that the sequencing of these events has a much greater effect on females' marital stability than on that of males. For example, in the sequence where marriage precedes first job, almost 86% of the males are found to be

TABLE 10.1. Staying Married for Males by Cross-Institutional and Institutional Sequences

Cross-Institutional Sequence	% Staying Married	Institutional Sequence	% Staying Married
Job–marriage	88.4	Marriage–child	89.2
		Child–marriage	86.6
		Child=marriage	83.6
Marriage–job	85.9	Marriage–child	86.5
		Child–marriage	73.7
		Child=marriage	87.5
Job=marriage	83.8	Marriage–child	84.7
		Child–marriage	75.0
		Child=marriage	80.0

TABLE 10.2. Staying Married for Females by Cross-Institutional and Institutional Sequences

Cross-Institutional Sequence	% Staying Married	Institutional Sequence	% Staying Married
Job–marriage	86.6	Marriage–child	88.4
		Child–marriage	70.4
		Child=marriage	82.6
Marriage–job	77.2	Marriage–child	79.3
		Child–marriage	67.7
		Child=marriage	71.0
Job=marriage	81.5	Marriage–child	83.3
		Child–marriage	71.4
		Child=marriage	70.4

still married, compared to about 77% of the females.[2] In regard to institutional sequencing, gender differences also exist. One such consistent gender difference is that female marital stability is more negatively affected by premarital births for all levels of cross-institutional sequences than is the marital stability for males, though both genders are negatively affected by premarital births. One reason for these gender differences may be that the females experiencing premarital births may have been much younger when married than their male counterparts. That is, the young males may not have received the pressure to marry in such cases to the degree that the young females were expected to marry.

Tables 10.3 and 10.4 contain the log-linear coefficients (lambda) for the estimated effects of cross-institutional sequences, institutional sequences, and the covariate of age at marriage. In order to keep the log-linear model in a relatively simple form, institutional and cross-

TABLE 10.3. Estimated Coefficients for the Effects of Cross-Institutional Sequences, Institutional Sequences, and Age at Marriage on Males Staying Married

Variable	Lambda	*SE*	*z*
Constant	.845	.035	24.01
Cross-institutional	–.046	.031	–1.47
Institutional	–.094	.029	–3.24
Age at marriage	–.182	.025	–7.24

Note. $L^2 = 2.72$, $p = .605$.

TABLE 10.4. Estimated Coefficients for the Effects of Cross-Institutional Sequences, Institutional Sequences, and Age at Marriage on Females Staying Married

Variable	Lambda	*SE*	*z*
Constant	.743	.027	26.94
Cross-institutional	–.093	.023	–3.99
Institutional	–.176	.025	–6.96
Age at marriage	–.168	.024	–6.87

Note. $L^2 = 3.621$, $p = .460$.

institutional sequences are collapsed into two values. The two values for cross-institutional sequences are either (1) job-marriage or (2) marriage-job and job=marriage. For the institutional sequences, values are collapsed into either (1) marriage–child or (2) child–marriage and child=marriage. In addition, age at marriage is collapsed into two categories: those marrying at the age of 20 or younger, and those marrying at the age of 21 or older. This coding allows for a relatively clear interpretation of effect coefficients as contributions of deviant sequences or normative sequences and age at marriage.

A comparison between Tables 10.3 and 10.4 further highlights gender differences. For instance, when age at marriage is a covariate for males staying married, cross-institutional sequences do not have a statistically significant effect. For males the single most important variable in the model is age at marriage, whereas for females age at marriage is slightly less important than deviance from the institutional sequence. For females, cross-institutional sequences continue to have a significant effect on staying married, despite the addition of the covariate age at marriage.

Both institutional deviance and cross-institutional deviance have a greater effect on females' marital stability than on males' marital stability.

This section demonstrates that sequencing deviance has negative effects on marital stability for both males and females. When the covariate age at marriage is considered, the effects for both cross-institutional and institutional sequencing deviance remain for females' marital stability, but the cross-institutional sequencing is no longer statistically significant for males. The importance of institutional deviance for females' marital stability is placed in perspective by the finding that institutional deviance has a slightly greater effect on females' marital stability than does age at marriage.

Deviance Measured with the Career Conformity Scale

This second section of the data analysis is concerned with the effects for the joint career deviance on marital stability. That is, the focus is on neither the institutional sequences nor the cross-institutional sequences; rather, it is on the combined career deviance for both. In this analysis, the effects of career deviance for various orderings of first job, first marriage, and first child are examined by means of the CCS.

Tables 10.5 and 10.6 show that career deviance has a statistically

TABLE 10.5. Probit Regression for Males' Age at Marriage and CCS Score with Staying Married

Variable	Regression coefficient	*SE*	Coeff./*SE*
Intercept	4.849	0.172	28.21
Age at marriage	0.042	0.007	5.98
CCS score	0.002	0.001	2.59

Note. χ^2 = 3,844.86, *df.* = 3,739.

TABLE 10.6. Probit Regression for Females' Age at Marriage and CCS Score with Staying Married

Variable	Regression coefficient	*SE*	Coeff./*SE*
Intercept	4.294	0.168	25.51
Age at marriage	0.058	0.008	7.15
CCS score	0.006	0.001	6.50

Note. χ^2 = 3,669.86, *df.* = 3,562.

significant ($p < .05$) negative effect on the probability of staying married. Conversely, the greater the career conformity to the modal pattern (job–marriage–child), the greater the probability of staying married. The effect of career conformity is almost three times higher for females than for males. This is consistent with the findings in the first section of the data analysis that both institutional and cross-institutional sequences have a greater effect on females' marital stability than on males' marital stability.

DISCUSSION

The findings are fairly clear. Males' marital stability is negatively affected by institutional deviance but not by cross-institutional deviance when early life events are used to measure career deviance. Females' marital stability is negatively affected by both institutional and cross-institutional deviance; however, it is much more strongly affected by institutional than by cross-institutional deviance. When both forms of deviance are combined into the CCS, the pattern is confirmed: Females have a regression coefficient three times that for the males. From the event sequence analysis in Table 10.4 that partitions this effect for females, it is clear that although a large part of the deviance is a result of premarital births (institutional deviance), there is a significant effect for deviance in sequencing first job and first marriage (cross-institutional deviance).

The general picture these data portray is that females who follow the normative sequence for first job, first marriage, and first child have a lower probability of marital disruptions later in life. The impact for premarital births is expected and has been previously noted by Morgan and Rindfuss (1985). The interesting effect is the cross-institutional one in a culture that is just turning the corner in terms of women's entering the labor force in large numbers. That is, there appears to be a significant effect for whether or not a woman marries before beginning her first job. In this regard, it would seem that work norms may have changed more quickly than family norms and will probably continue to do so.

These findings have important theoretical implications. First, the hypothesis that deviance is more of an individual or family trait can be examined in light of these data. If deviance is a general trait, then there would be an expected association between deviance in the sequencing of early life events and later marital disruption. Indeed, this association exists. The question that is posed at the outset of this chapter is whether the association represents one between causal variables (early life sequencing deviance) and an effect variable (marital disruptions), or whether it represents two expressions (early career deviance and marital disruptions) of one common trait of deviance. It is critical for the theory of family development that this question be resolved. The other interpretation for this association is the trait interpretation, which would rely on a genetic theory of social systems. Although such a theory only exists in rudimentary form, such as in sociobiology, it nonetheless poses a real alternative to the ecological approach.

If career deviance and marital disruptions are related through the common factor of deviance as a trait, then this trait should express itself in various areas such as work and family, regardless of the distinctions made by an ecological theory. In fact, the association between the CCS and marital disruption would support this view, but with a major exception. That exception is that females' early career deviance is more strongly related to later marital instability than is males' early deviance. From a genetic point of view, this leaves the unlikely hypothesis that females express more deviance than males in various ways. This seems an unlikely and untenable perspective.

Even more doubt is cast on the genetic or trait interpretation when the partitioned effects are examined. For both males and females, there is a substantial difference between the cross-institutional and institutional effects on marital stability. However, the cross-institutional effects are statistically significant for females but not for males. Again, this leaves the trait interpretation with the unlikely interpretation that females express deviance in more areas.

The approach taken here views these differences as caused by the differential norms or rules that each gender is expected to follow in regard to career sequencing. Because norms are separated into those appropriate for both genders and those appropriate to only one gender, certain sequences are normative for one gender and deviant for the other gender. For example, although a premarital birth has statistically significant effects for both genders, it clearly has a larger effect for females. The fact that males and females follow different norms in some institutional areas implies that the cross-institutional norms must also be different for each gender, since the different institutional sequences must be coordinated between institutions for males in a different way than for females. This explains the finding in this study that females' marital stability is affected by the sequencing of first job and first marriage, whereas males' marital stability is not significantly affected by this sequencing.

One last implication of this analysis is that when a dependent variable is clearly within a particular institution such as the family, cross-institutional deviance has less effect on that variable than does within-institution deviance. This implies that deviance from the norms within an institution has the greatest effect on both other norms within that institution and behavior in that institution. So, for example, both males' and females' early career deviance in the institution of the family has a greater effect on marital stability than does cross-institutional sequencing. However, this conclusion must be a guarded one, since the event of a premarital birth in North American society continues to carry a good deal of normative weight in regard to sanctions and timing of other life events. These results could also reflect this particularly salient event.

CONCLUSION

This chapter offers a perspective on change that requires the identification of the type of change one is considering: developmental change, evolutionary change, or random change. In developmental change, a unit of analysis (be it family or institution) changes structure and norms so as to be considered in a qualitatively different state or stage than was previously the case. Evolutionary change is more continuous than the discrete changes involved in developmental processes. Evolutionary change has two principal forms, adaptation (natural selection) and mutation. The major way in which institutions change is adaptation.

Besides identification of the type of change, the study of change also demands the specification of the level of analysis. This is not to say that change does not involve complex interactions between levels; it does. However, the study of change must start by distinguishing the changes at each level before moving to such complex analyses.

The two principal ways in which the norms of an institution change are institutional deviance and cross-institutional adaptation. Institutional deviance refers to the failure of individuals or groups to conform to the normative structure of one particular institution. The most important form of this deviance is that in which some other institution's norms fail to coordinate with the norms of the first institution, and people or groups conform to one institution but are deviant in the other. In a sense, people and families must choose between different sets of norms from different institutions. It is important to note that this form of deviance is analyzed as aggregated behavior of individuals or groups.

Cross-institutional adaptation is where two institutions align their timing and sequencing norms so as to bring them into better synchronization. This form of adaptation is usually the result of traumas in the system, experienced by individuals and groups as high stress loads because too many events and transitions are occurring simultaneously or in a sequence that creates stress. These events, from at least two different institutions, are nonetheless normative. In this case, the norms are not contrary to one another and do not require choice, as with institutional deviance. Rather, with cross-institutional deviance, following all the norms results in such traumas as mass family breakdown or mental illness. For example, the normative sequence for females of completing school, starting a first job, getting married, and then having a child may create immense stress as each institution's demands for time and competence increase. So females remain in school longer, perhaps until 25 years of age, as expectations for "higher education" increase in strength. Females may then find it increasingly time-consuming to move from the contract work of secondary employment to the benefit and promotionable arena of primary employment as the years race by them. Courtship and marriage may take longer as achievements in education and work create "marriage squeeze" problems in mate availability. Finally, these sequencing norms have added so much stress, in terms of the increasing level of performance standards associated with each step in the sequence, that female fertility and perhaps fecundity are bound to suffer. This is an example of the buildup of stress and trauma over a period of time while individuals are following noncontradictory and commonly held cross-institutional sequencing norms. Clearly, the reasons for deviance from cross-institutional sequencing and timing norms may be more closely tied to trauma and aggregate pathology than would be true of institutional deviance. This is because the cross-institutional sequencing norms appear to be consistent and possible, in sharp contrast to the contradictions between institutional norms that are associated with institutional deviance.

One last point needs to be made in regard to institutional change by means of institutional deviance and cross-institutional adaptation. In institutional deviance, as the deviant behavior becomes more frequent, the sanctions at the group level begin to change. Thus, with institutional deviance, behavioral change precedes changes in sanctions.

NOTES

1. Note that positive sanctions can be regarded as the inverse of negative sanctions, so there is no need for a separate dimension for the strength of positive sanctions in addition to the strength of negative sanctions.

2. Note that in the Family History Survey, all females (not just the subset in this chapter) reported more divorces than did males. This is probably due to the fact that females marry earlier and live longer than do males, so the female

respondents had more years at risk than the males did, and more survived to report. It is also probably true that females who work have higher rates of divorce than females who do not, and hence the subsample used in this chapter would have reported more divorces than the males did. Unfortunately, the data set does not contain data on whether males' wives were employed, so this corresponding group is not available for comparison.

PART IV

CONCLUSIONS

CHAPTER 11

Family Dynamics: A Second Look

The purposes of this chapter are (1) to reformulate and summarize the theory of family development in light of the preceding chapters, and (2) to address the issue of defining stages of family development. Defining stages of family development has been left until this point because event research can be conducted without the specification of stages. However, there can be no real theoretical progress without a solution to this problem of stage specification, because the theoretical meanings of event analyses are derived from the inferences to stages of family development.

SUMMARY OF MAJOR POINTS

First, I briefly summarize some of the major points in the previous chapters.

Some developmentalists may have believed that families developed in a rigid, lockstep way. The present work argues against an assumption that the order of stages in family development is invariant and that developmental tasks for a stage have to be met before a family can move to the next stage. In the research presented here, we see that the probability of a transition is not linear and monotonic. Rather, the probability of a transition to another stage appears to be based on the present stage the family occupies and the duration of time it has spent in that stage. The sequencing norms for the family are largely responsible for the stage dependence, while the timing norms for the family largely establish the duration dependence for a transition to another stage.

Although the process of development is defined by the duration and stage dependence for the probability of a transition, that does not mean that duration and stage are uniformly significant for all levels of analysis, or for all variables other than the probability of a transition (e.g., Menaghan, 1983). For example, in the analysis of dyadic relationships (Chapter 8), the stage a dyad occupies seems more important in regard to relationship variables than does the duration in the stage. Whether or not this is true of other relationships, such as those of parent–child and siblings, remains unanswered. Indeed, it may be that throughout the process of development stage is a better predictor than duration in stage, though this has yet to be determined.

The dynamic aspects of the theory of family development focus on predicting the stages in the process from the present stage the family occupies and the duration in that stage. In the language of cause and effect,[1] this means that the stages can be either independent variables or dependent variables in this system. For example, based on the present family stage and the duration of time in that stage, the prediction might be that there is a low probability for a transition to another stage and that families in such a stage have a high probability of remaining in that stage. For example, childless couples who have been married for 30 years would tend to remain childless.

Despite the fact that the major focus of the dynamic analysis is on predicting the probabilities for stage transitions, this stochastic aspect is not the sole content of the theory. Almost all researchers and theorists have identified variables that are correlated with the family stage, such as marital satisfaction. However, this associational research is often confronted by threats to its validity from other time-related variables, such as cohort, period, and age effects. Despite these threats, the correlates of various stages are of great interest. "Does communication in the marital dyad change by family stage?" is an example of this type of question.

Although it is admittedly interesting to examine the correlates of various stages, the research presented here has asked a different type of question, oriented toward the *dynamic* nature of family development. What I have pursued is the question of whether or not family career paths and cross-institutional paths are associated with events in later life, such as marital disruptions. This area of research is correlational rather than stochastic in exactly the same sense that the research on correlates of family stages is; however, it attempts to capture more of the dynamic character of family development than the stage-oriented research has done. It must be noted, nevertheless, that this research is subject to the same threats to its validity as the stage-oriented research.

As families and relationships develop, they create a path or career history. The research presented in Chapter 9 has found that although men and women share the same modal career for early life events, there is evidence for gender-specific sequencing norms. Furthermore, these gender-specific norms seem to vary by the period of time in which one is socialized and marries. Childbearing is largely responsible for the gender differences; yet the timing of childbearing and its position in the sequence of other events cannot be attributed to biological gender differences. Many of the changes in career patterns over time are related to changes in other norms, such as those regulating family size, age at first birth, and women's entry and participation in the labor force.

Institutional norms appear to be stronger in effect than do cross-institutional norms. Undoubtedly this is difficult to determine, since these norms are seldom independent. However, it seems that sequences of family events have a stronger effect on marital stability than do cross-institutional sequences. This may also attest to the fact that the dependent variable of marital stability is clearly within the institution of marriage and the family, rather than work or educational institutions.

Following Modell (1980), I have suggested that behavioral changes in the form of deviance from existing timing and sequencing norms precede changes in normative expectations. In part this is a logical proposition, given that norms as rules must have at least some adherence or they will no longer be considered rules. However, a more important point must be stressed: When normative sequences or timing norms in an institution such as the family are not coordinated with timing and sequencing norms in other institutions, some of these norms must shift if society is to continue to operate in a relatively systematic and organized fashion. The way in which those norms are brought into alignment is through systematic nonconformity to some of those norms. The term "*systematic* nonconformity" (as opposed to random variation) means not only deviation from one set of norms, but deviation in a specific direction, to permit greater conformity to the sequencing and timing norms of other institutions. When the deviant behavior becomes modal, we can say that the process of a change to new sequencing and timing norms is complete. It must be remembered that these sequencing and timing norms supply the reason why the probabilities for transitions depend upon stage and duration in the stage.

All of the points made above leave us with one very obvious question: "What then produces the conditions that put previously aligned and articulated cross-institutional timing and sequencing norms out of alignment?" This question really asks for the sources of social change above the cross-institutional and institutional levels. Another way to view this is that within any social system we can analyze the following levels:

Individual
Relationship
Group (family and other groups)
Institutional (family, work, education, religion, polity)
Cross-institutional (family–work, work–education, etc.)

However, once we move beyond the cross-institutional level, the society (e.g., the United States or Canada) or culture (e.g., North America) can no longer be the focus of the discussion. The focus changes to analyzing those cross-cultural processes and changes taking place in the world system and their influence on the normative fabric of any given society. This task is beyond the scope of the present work.

STAGE SPECIFICATION

The specification of a set of theoretical stages is not the only problem confronting the theory of family development, but it is one of the most important and central problems. As we have seen, research can continue using events to indicate stage transition points, even though we are unclear as to the nature of the stage being indicated. This approach is fraught with difficulties for the theory, even though it is a workable strategy for empirical research. The theoretical problem is that we have no way to accumulate theoretical knowledge about stage transitions unless we can specify the stages.

Criticisms of Previous Stage Conceptions

The concept of stages of the family has been criticized by many scholars—for example, Schram (1979) and Nock (1979). Borne and his associates (1979) list five reasons for these various critiques. Although the majority of reasons listed by Borne et al. (1979) are methodological in nature, two of these criticisms have theoretical implications. Borne et al. say that the theory has failed to explain much of the variance in such dependent variables as communication and marital satisfaction, and that the stages specified fail to tap into the truly important aspects of family life. The second criticism suggests that the stage conceptions in use have little *validity*, and the first criticism suggests that the stage conceptions in use offer little if any *predictive value*. From a theoretical perspective, it seems that any theory should be able to make claims in these two areas. So these criticisms cannot be treated lightly.

These criticisms of the stage concept are largely accurate; however, the reasons why are quite complex. Generally, the criticisms are true because the concept of stages evolved not from the theory as much as from a normative description of families in North America during the 1940s and 1950s. In order to understand how this has misdirected this component of the theory, it is important to examine in some detail the theoretical rather than methodological problems with the concept.

1. There has long been a confusion as to whether family stages are derived and generated from axioms in the theory, or whether they may be developed ad hoc by a researcher for a particular research question. If family stages are ad hoc then we should not expect them to reflect the theory as much as the interest and limitations in the empirical research. For example, Rodgers (1973) states:

> These classifications are not real but imposed on the family by the researcher in order to make comparisons which he considers important. Thus, different categories may be used for different problems; that is, the family career may be broken up in various ways for various purposes. (p. 78)

Although Rodgers is discussing the operationalization of the stages concept, this statement nonetheless gives more license to researchers than it does guidance as to appropriate ways to divide up the family career into family stages.

2. This brings up the point that the criteria for family stages have not been theoretically derived or theoretically justified. For example, Aldous (1978, pp. 83–86) discusses the myriad of criteria scholars have used to determine family stages. Among these criteria are changes in family membership, the individual developmental stages of the oldest child, and the age range of the children. Indeed, Aldous herself adopts the two criteria of school placement of the oldest child and discontinuance of work careers (1978, p. 86). From the perspective of this book, the criterion of school placement relates to a cross-institutional event, as does that of work discontinuance. Neither of these is clearly a family event. Furthermore, there is no attempt to demonstrate why these criteria are theoretically justified.

3. Because stage conceptions have been treated as ad hoc constructions and not tied to a set of theoretical definitions and axioms, there exists a plethora of stage conceptions in both the theoretical and empirical literature. For instance, Aldous (1978) presents four different stage conceptions ranging from one containing five stages to one containing seven. In the empirical literature, we find studies using from eight stages

(Rollins & Feldman, 1970) to four stages (Anderson et al., 1983) to examine the same dependent variable, marital satisfaction.

4. In all these diverse stage conceptions, there is one common element: Events such as the wedding day or the start of elementary school are used to construct the stage. However, no careful definition of the relationship between events and stages exists. Indeed, the exact relationship between events and stages is unclear. For example, Aldous (1978, p. 81) states that events are not points in time as much as variable periods of time. However, she defines a stage as a qualitatively distinct period in the life of a family. So the question remains: "How can a *qualitatively distinct* period have a *quantitatively gradual* transition point?" Furthermore, if such a position were adopted by the theory, it would mean that the computation of time spent within a stage is at least as variable as the duration of gradual events demarcating that stage. This would make the entire conception of family stages rather useless from both a theoretical and a methodological standpoint.

5. Stages of family development have often been criticized because they have systematically excluded certain family forms, such as single-parent families and childless couples. Not only have the stage conceptions not exhausted the possible family forms within North America, but they have failed to have the cross-cultural applicability required of a social-scientific theory. That is, it is commonly understood that one characteristic of a good scientific theory is that it attempts not to be myopically rooted in one culture or one particular period of history, so that its applicability and scope are not arbitrarily restricted. For example, many stage conceptions use the divisions of children's elementary and secondary school attendance for demarcating stages (Aldous, 1978, pp. 85–86). Naturally, not all cultures use these divisions, and not all children are required to attend secondary school. These categories are neither universally applicable in the present nor useful in historical analyses, so that we could compare family career sequences using the same set of stages for different historical periods.

6. A similar criticism to the preceding is that not only do stage conceptions fail to offer an exhaustive set of stages that have applicability across cultures and historical periods; many of the stage conceptions also fail to meet the simple logical criterion of being mutually exclusive. That is, when we discuss a set of possible stages, it is usually taken for granted that no two stages can be occupied simultaneously. However, stage conceptions such as Duvall's (1971) fail to meet this criterion. For instance, it is quite possible that a family may simultaneously contain children who are infants (Duvall's Stage II) and adolescents (Duvall's Stage V). The selection of only the oldest child as the determining factor

does little except to weight one member of the family unduly and to conceal the variation in families without theoretical justification.

7. Finally, there is confusion regarding the level of analysis to which the concept of stage belongs. For example, some authors assume that the age (maturation and development) of a key individual such as the oldest child is a key element in determining a family stage. However, others suggest that roles and role relationships are the key elements in family stages. Finally, Aldous asks us to "[n]ote that the concept *critical role transitions,* refers to individuals while *morphogenesis,* and *stage* refer to families" (1978, p. 81). Clearly, there is some need for clarity in regard to the relationship between levels of analysis and stages.

These criticisms serve to point out the criteria that any conception of stages should meet. These criteria are as follows:

1. The set of stages should be exhaustive of the possible family forms both within and between cultures and time periods.
2. The set of stages should be mutually exclusive, so that no two stages may be occupied simultaneously.
3. The set of stages should be systematically related to the basic definitions and assumptions of the theory.
   a. The set of stages should be theoretically and systematically related to the concept of events.
   b. The set of stages should be theoretically and systematically related to levels of analysis.

Morphological Stages

Many scholars have used simple changes in the membership of the family group (e.g., the addition of a second child, children leaving home, or the death of a spouse) to indicate stages of the family group. Indeed, Aldous (1978) suggests that these changes in group structure be termed "morphogenesis," a term denoting changes in structure. This structural perspective, when joined with the concepts of domicile (space) and events (time), supplies a concept of stages that meets the criteria discussed above.

Returning to earlier statements of the theory of family development, such as those by Aldous (1978) and Rodgers (1973), is a good way to begin. Aldous (1978, p. 80) views stages as qualitatively distinct periods in the life course of the family. Rodgers (1973) believes that stages are unique configurations of roles and role relationships. These are helpful insights when we reconsider the nature of positions and roles. In Chapter 9, I have stated that a position in a social structure is similar to a point in geometry; that is, it has no content and simply locates nodes of the structure. Those familiar with kinship analysis will be familiar with this type of thinking. Indeed, the group structure of the family is largely a kinship structure. Recall that in Chapter 3, the family as a group is mainly defined by the presence of a parent–child relation. This is a structural definition, since the social roles for a parent and a child and for the parent–child relationship change from culture to culture. The family group therefore is defined as a structure that, at a minimum, includes both a consanguineal and a generational relation. Although it is not analytically necessary to identify gender in addition to consanguinity and generation as part of the structure, a case can be made that social roles and norms are so gender-specific in all cultures as to warrant the inclusion of gender relations in family structure, and hence in stages of the family. Family stages, then, must be stages relevant to the development of this group structure. Thus, we can imagine many family stages based upon family structures. For example, a single-parent family is a minimal structure perhaps developed from the divorce of a previous member. A family with five children is much farther from the minimal structure.

As with all abstractions, when we decide to observe or measure stages, we need to set spatial boundaries. In regard to the structure of the family, it is important to remember that the positions in a structure will be governed by norms that establish the social role for each position for any given culture. In addition, the role relationships between actors occupying positions are constituted by norms. A simple example of a fairly universal norm is that forbidding incest between a parent and a child. This norm is only one among the many that govern this role relationship. The social roles and role relationships for a family usually take place within a specific environment, such as a domicile or several domiciles. The physical relations for most family interaction are established when one is "in" or "out" of the family domicile. Furthermore, these physical relations are too often interpreted as meaning "boundaries," implying that the family only exists within these parameters. It is more appropriate to use domicile boundaries to establish the spatial relationships of members, so that being "in" or "out" of the boundaries is a form of relationship captured by our stages concept. In addition, these boundaries, like social roles, change from culture to culture. So the abstract concept of "domicile" defines the spatial relations for the family, but the measurement definition of domicile must change from culture to culture. In regard to stages of family development, the spatial relations are most useful in determining the composition of a stage. The domicile provides a sense of spatial relations in cases where it is equally valuable information whether children are residing within or outside of the domicile.

Thus far, it appears that family stages can simply be constructed by the combination of positional structures and spatial relations. However, such a structural understanding of family stages is very misleading, because it neglects the role of institutional norms in establishing stages for family development. For example, the group structure of a marriage and a cohabiting couple can be said to be identical; that is, both are mixed-gender dyads. However, as the empirical studies in Chapters 7 and 8 have demonstrated, there are quite different transition probabilities and effects on dyadic measures for these two types of dyads. Furthermore, certain institutional transitions (e.g., divorce) can only be experienced in marriages. What, in fact, set these two dyadic structures apart are the institutional norms appropriate for each. Indeed, many people cohabit precisely because they do *not* want the institutional norms and roles of marriage.

How do we incorporate this notion of institutional norms with the idea of group structure to form a more adequate concept of family stages? It is important to recall that a stage is a qualitatively distinct period in the life of a family that is bounded by transition events. The institutional norms are applied only to those structural units that have experienced these transition events. For example, the static norms regarding matrimonial inheritance and property apply only to those who are married. Regardless of current "palimony" cases, these formal norms have not been fully applied to cohabitation. The event that separates one set of norms for cohabitation from the other set of norms for marriage is the event of the wedding. Thus, in order to capture the interaction between group structure and institutional norms, the idea of "transition events" must be added to our concept of family stages.

Although the idea of transition events being tied to group positional structure may appear somewhat foreign, in reality it is not. However, in order to understand the intimate connection between kinship positions and transition events, we must closely examine kinship position terms. In the study of kinship, a position in a family or kinship group is defined by three relations: (1) generation, (2) affinal or consanguineal bonds, and (3) gender. For example, the position of "mother" is one generation ascending from "ego," a consanguineal relation, and female gender. From these three relations, the essential kinship positions can be generated. Schusky (1965, p. 8) lists the basic ones as father, mother, brother, sister, husband, wife, daughter, and son. A close examination of the husband–wife positional relationship shows that transition events are important in defining these positional terms. For example, Schusky (1965, p. 5) defines the affinal relation as a "marital bond." If this is strictly interpreted, then a cohabiting couple is only related through a common domicile and not through an affinal relationship. The positions of husband and wife are then defined as follows: "A husband is a married male" and "A wife is a married female." However, it is clear from this definition that a married person is one who has been "wed"—that is, one who has entered the specific relationship of marriage, which has been acknowledged by the rite of passage or event of a wedding. So the kinship positional structures already contain elements of transition events in the definitions of the positions.

Group structure and family norms interact to form family stages in two ways. First, the group structure supplies incumbents for the positions. These incumbents are the necessary material for the application of the static norms. These static norms construct the family roles *within* a stage of the family life course. In order for the norms and roles to be operational, there must be an actor or incumbent in a position. The second way in which norms and structure interact is much more interesting. The processual, institutional norms apply to a specific structure and suggest the normative transition event and the next group structure. Thus, early marriage is often accompanied by the question "When will the first child arrive?" The arrival of the first child is the event that marks the transition to a parental structure and the stage of new parenthood. A stage transition is indicated by a change in group structure and in the relationship of the group to the boundaries of the domicile.

The concept of "family stage," then, is defined by three elements: (1) the group positional structure, expressed in universal kinship terms (Schusky, 1965); (2) a transition event, which divides the previous stage's positional structure from the next stage's positional structure; and (3) the spatial relationship of being within or outside of the domicile.

A more clear idea of this definition of family stages in terms of structure, event, and domicile is afforded by examining the normative pattern in North America. Most families begin as marriages. Although a marriage is *not* a family group, it clearly is a stage in family development because the processual norms define it as such. Most family groups begin with the structure of two adult members and one child. For most families, the next structural transition is the addition of another child. The change to this two-child structure adds the sibling roles and relationship. Although more children may not add any more social relationships, the structure and, by definition, the stage of the family change with each addition. The structure of the average family changes again as children leave the domicile to begin their own lives. Some children may leave the nest for a few years and then return for a few years. Every time there is a change in structure in relation to the spatial boundary of the domicile, there is a stage transition. The final structural stage transition may be the last child's final departure from the domicile; at this point, there is no longer a family group within the domicile because of the absence of a generational consanguineal bond (parent–child). This is not to say that this, like early marriage, is not a family stage. To reiterate, family stage is defined as the interaction of domicile, group structure, and institutional norms as indicated by transition events, not simply by the group structure. Hence, the family group may cease to exist within the domicile, but the family stage does not necessarily cease to exist; the "empty nest" marriage does constitute a stage. The concept of family stage is, therefore, a much broader concept than that of the family as a group.

Several authors (e.g., White & Reid, 1984; Eichler, 1988) have suggested some conventions for diagramming structurally defined stages. Eichler's approach has much to recommend it; however, she does not adopt traditional kinship diagramming conventions (Schusky, 1965). The more usual way of diagramming kinship structures is already embedded in a body of knowledge and theory (e.g., H. C. White, 1963). Figure 11.1 shows what some of the more familiar family stages look like when a traditional kinship approach similar to Eichler's is used.

Although this definition of family stages based on changes in family structure, domicile, and events is largely compatible with previous conceptions of family stages, it is not identical to these earlier conceptions. For instance, many previous scholars have relied on characteristics such as the ages of the children for delineating stages. The structural approach relies on the presence of incumbents in the positions alone. The reason for this should be clear: At the family or group level of analysis, the structure of the group is what is important. We do not want to confuse variables at the group level with variables at the relationship level (or family subunit level). For example, the relationship between a mother and a child continues to develop over time. This development is properly studied at the relationship level as a series of changes in the qualitative dimensions (stages) of that *relationship*. It is a mistake, however, to assume that it should be studied as a series of changes in the qualitative dimensions of the group. The major dimension of the group is its positional structure. The positional structure determines which roles and role relationships are available to actors. It is this dimension that defines the stages of the group, and not the stages of various family relationships, which should properly be studied at the relationship level.

Another potential area of conflict is the identification of how changes in structure take place. Aldous (1978, p. 81) suggests that changes in structure come about through changes in individuals, followed by changes in interaction patterns, followed by changes in group behavior patterns. This view, and others that attempt to explain changes in group structure as resulting from either the ontogenetic maturation of

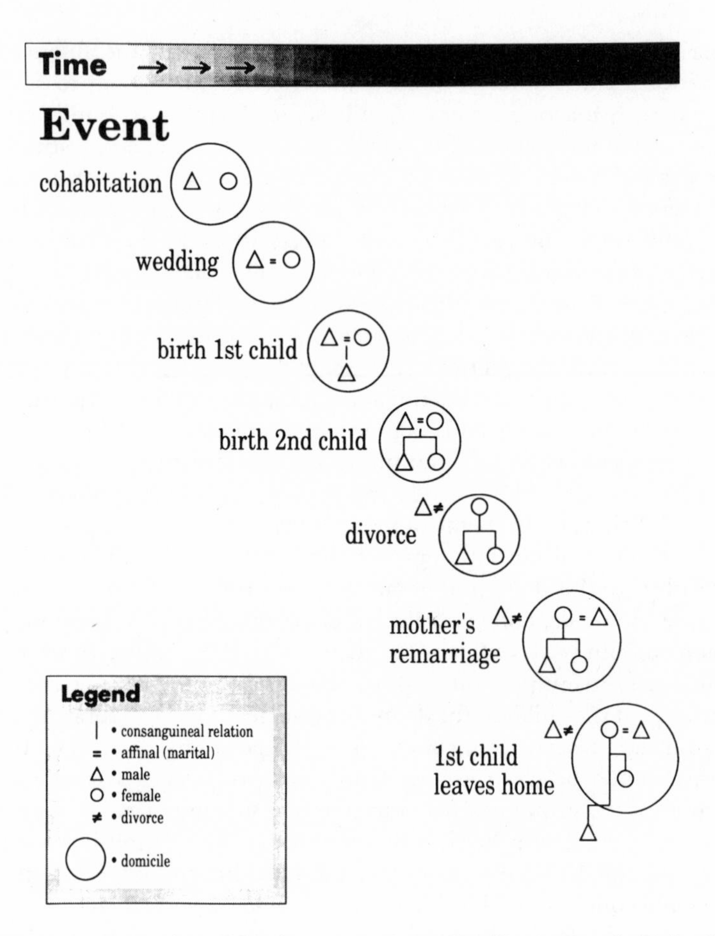

FIGURE 11.1. Examples of family stages. From *Families in Canada Today* (2nd ed., p. 26) by M. Eichler, 1988, Toronto: Gage. Copyright 1988 by Gage Educational Publishing Company. Adapted by permission.

the individual or the social maturation of the individual, have a difficult time explaining why there exists such uniformity in patterns of family development within a culture. If the causes for morphogenesis were ontogenetic, then the only explanation for cross-cultural difference would be gene pool differences or mutations. For example, the Kaingang in Brazil have no word or institution similar to "marriage" (Henry, 1964). If group structure were to develop from the ontogenetic progress of individuals, then it would seem that the difference between the Kaingang and North American is a genetic one. However, this seems a totally unacceptable argument.

On the other hand, the argument that individual maturation and interaction cause changes in group structure is equally problematic. If this were the case, why then would we find pervasive patterns of family development? Given the diversity of individuals, their ages, and their interaction patterns in families, could we really expect societal patterns of behavior to emerge from individual interactions in a relatively uniform and consistent manner?

The view that seems most compatible with morphogenesis is that a myriad of variables, both within and external to a family, affect the family. However, social-institutional norms are what largely account for the uniformity of family development. Furthermore, deviations from the institutional norms can often be explained by conformity to the norms of other social institutions, such as work or education. It seems more probable that the larger social system affects the smaller ones—in other words, that institutions affect group structure—than that individuals cause group changes, which then create uniformities in social systems.

The task of weighing this conception of family stages against others eventually falls on each individual scholar. The least that can be done here is to cite a few of the major strengths of this approach.

1. The structural approach gives a relatively clear definition of family stages that can easily be applied in cross-cultural research. This has not been a strength of previous stage conceptions.

2. The structural approach defines stages so that a family can only be in one stage at a time (mutually exclusive) and so that all possible stages can be generated (space-exhaustive). It is impossible to construct theory, models, and data without at least meeting the constraints of mutually exclusive categories that are exhaustive (i.e., countable).[2]

3. The structural–event approach allows for clarity at the group level of analysis and for the inclusion of the concept of events. It clearly distinguishes between a family group and a marital group, while acknowledging that family institutional norms construct each as stages of family development. Furthermore, this approach allows for the distinction among marriage as a group, marriage as a stage, and marriage as one of the relationships within a family (the sibling relationship and the parent–child relationship are others).

4. The structural approach fits well with other studies of groups in sociology and with other studies of kinship.

5. Another advantage to this approach to family stages is that for any set number of positions (say, two to four), a finite set of stages can be generated. This generation of a possibility space for family stages allows for the development of some rather interesting measures of family development, such as entropy. This is discussed in the next section of this chapter.

6. Lastly, the structural approach straightens out some of the previous confusion among the development of family relationships (relationship level), the development of the family (group level), and stages of family development (interaction between group structure and normative events).

Entropy and the Strength of Family Norms

A set of theoretical stages for family development that meets the criteria of mutually exclusive and exhaustive categories allows for some progress in the analysis of change in populations. For example, we could identify all the possible stages that any family of a given size might occupy. If we imagine that this set of n stages (states) is unconstrained by any other variables, then the probability of any state is $1/n$. However, we already know that of the vast number of possible family structural stages, only a relatively small number of them occur with much frequency. A cross-sectional view of the population of families at different ages would show that families in the first 3 years tend to occupy only one or two stages in any significant numbers. Families that are between 15 and 20 years old show a much greater diversity of stages. Many of these families have had the time to experience events that construct different structural stages, such as divorce, remarriage, and death of a spouse. The overall picture, then, is that as families age, stages become more diversified. Although for any one family the process may be one of beginning, expansion, constriction, and ending, it may be a somewhat different type of process at the population level.[3]

The population process for families can be described by the degree to which the probability for stages departs from the random distribution. Thus, this process can be described by an "entropy" measure, such as that developed in the study of molecules. Although many scholars have made much of the philosophical implications of the concept of entropy (e.g., Prigogine & Stengers, 1984), the concept as used here is a strictly methodological one: Entropy is a measure of the degree of randomness in a distribution of frequencies for states. This measure is defined for a simple case of two disjoint states as follows:

$$e_i^n = \log \left[\binom{n}{i} \right] \quad (1)$$

where n = number of elements in the population
i = number of elements in a state
(Kemeny, Mirkil, Snell, & Thompson, 1958, p. 94)

This simple measure can be expanded to accommodate a much larger set of states and has applications to Markov processes (e.g., Kemeny et al., 1959).

The interpretation of the entropy measure is quite straightforward. For example, when trials are independent and the number of cases is equally distributed among the number of states, then the entropy measure is maximum. On the other hand, if all the cases are only in one state at each point in time, the entropy measure is 0. In other words, an entropy score of 0 refers to a deterministic situation, and an entropy score of 1 refers to a random distribution. When distributions are examined over time, the process should be characterized by a degree of entropy ranging between complete randomness and strict determinism.

What are the implications of family entropy as a population process for the theory of family development? For example, what is the interpretation of the situation where, for each time point in the age of families, we find that a single but different stage has a probability equal to 1? This distribution would indicate a deterministic process. In other words, the normative definitions regarding stage transitions would be so strong as to allow no exceptions. This situation is, of course, unlikely except in the nursery rhyme referred to more than once in this book: "First comes love, then comes marriage, then comes Suzie with a baby carriage." But this example demonstrates that entropy can be a meaningful measure of any family system's departure from strict normative determination on the one hand, or normlessness and chaos on the other hand. Regardless of culture, once we have a set of mutually exclusive and exhaustive theoretical stages, different cultures can be compared as to the degree of entropy in their family systems. A comparison of societies attempting to manage or control family size with societies encouraging fertility would be especially interesting.

Speculation on the Development of Stages

It is clear, both from the preceding chapters and from the discussion thus far in this chapter, that the concept of family stages is central for the theory of family development. It is also fairly clear that there are many different ways of approaching the study of family stages. For example, a family stage can be designated as the period between two events. The discussion above has gone to some length to tie the theoretical concepts of stage and event together. However, the various ways in which scholars have approached and measured stages seem to indicate that stages show a progression within a social system rather than simply that a myriad of approaches are possible. In Chapter 10, I have discussed the possibility of institutional development over time and concluded that not much is known about the ways in which social institutions develop internally. However, cross-institutional adaptation in order to synchronize the timing and sequencing of events between institutions is seen as a major component in institutional change. It is actually impossible to separate the extent to which institutional change is attributable to an institution's internal development and the extent to which it is attributable to cross-institutional adaptation. Regardless of the causes of these changes, however, it is possible to detect some of the elements in the institutional development of family stages.

Although the process of development within the institution of the family is usually slow and gradual, certain changes are nonetheless discernible. For instance, in the 1950s cohabitation was certainly not considered to be a stage of family development, or even a possible stage. In addition, divorce was perceived as a deviant event in family development, and certainly not as a marker for the beginning of a new stage of family development (Ahrons & Rodgers, 1987). The changes in how we perceive these events and stages are not simply the results of greater awareness and more extensive data reporting in the social sciences. Rather, the institution of the family as a set of social norms has changed.

In previous chapters, I have already discussed some of the elements of social-institutional change. For instance, I have stated that behavioral change precedes changes in social expectations. This is because a social norm comes into existence first as behavior, then as the expectation that there is a behavioral regularity. For example, the expectation that drivers will run yellow traffic lights is based more on behavioral regularities than on any moral feeling that drivers should or ought to run yellow traffic lights. However, once the behavioral regularity exists, then the expectations develop.

Behavioral changes may come about because of conformity to the norms of some other institution or because of a set of random historical events (e.g., war or pestilence). Clearly, different types of events may trigger a change in family structure. Some of these events are random or haphazard; other events, such as world economic pressures, are exogenous to a particular social system. Many such events can create changes in family structure, as did the loss of lives during World War II. However, these events must be seen as non-normative, historical events.

The events that are tied to the normatively defined transitions in the family can be more precisely termed "transition events." Thus, transition events are closely tied to institutional sequencing and timing norms. Random events may have effects on family structure, but these effects are neither "on time" nor "off time," because they are neither behavioral uniformities nor social expectations. It seems that as events become consistently tied to a transition to a specific group structure, the behavior pattern approaches greater frequency in the population until it finally becomes a modal pattern. For example, a premarital birth undoubtedly has a consequence on group structure, but it is clearly not a behavioral uniformity or an expectation. Cohabitation has become much more frequent in North America, and close to half of premarital cohabitations end in marriage. This has led some scholars to speculate that cohabitation is evolving into a stage of family development (Gwartney-Gibbs, 1986). However, at the present time it is not sufficiently frequent as an occurrence in the population to be considered an expected step toward marriage.

In the last century, longevity has sufficiently increased so as to allow many couples in North America more postparental years. Certainly, the postparental stage is a normatively defined stage, in that the norms dictate that the children leave the nest. However, the internal role expectations for the postparental stage remain somewhat amorphous: There are family institutional timing and sequencing norms, but few internal role expectations. This lack of internal role expectations can be seen most clearly when we compare the postparental stage to the family stage with two children. Clearly, a host of both formal and informal norms surround the duties and obligations in the family. By contrast, in the postparental stage, not all of these duties and obligations are entirely clear as yet. For instance, do children have a formal legal filial responsibility for the welfare of their parents?

Table 11.1 summarizes this discussion. What this table suggests is that family stages develop their complete institutional normative fabric only after a considerable time in the society. That is, time is needed for an event to become consistently tied to a group structure (Phase I to Phase II). If the event is not consistently tied to a group structure, then it is haphazard in its effect rather than uniform. Once the event and a specific group structure are consistently associated, then the behavior may become increasingly frequent (Phase II to Phase III). Such is the argument regarding the evolution of cohabitation as a family stage. Lastly, the

TABLE 11.1. Phases in the Development of Family Stages

Phases of stages	Determining criteria	Interpretive domain	Concepts	Example
Phase I	Transitional event	Historical (demographic)	Sequence timing	Premarital birth
Phase II	Transitional event Group structure	Historical Morphological	Sequence Timing Stage	Cohabitation
Phase III	Transitional event Group structure Modal behavior	Historical Morphological Sociological	Sequence Timing Stage Institutional norms	Postparental stage
Phase IV	Transitional event Group structure Modal behavior Expectations	Historical Morphological Sociological Psychological	Sequence Timing Stage Institutional norms Roles	Families with two children

frequently and consistently associated event and group structure, which are regulated by timing and sequencing norms, develop a set of norms attached to the positions in the group structure (roles). These role expectations represent the most fully developed family stage (Phase IV).

It should be clear that stages may evolve and devolve. For example, the stage for families with large numbers of children seems to be devolving in North America, while cohabitation and remarriage seem to be evolving. It is clear that some events and structures may move through some phases, but then reverse direction and devolve. The exact conditions that determine the evolution of family stages through these phases are constructed from a diverse set of variables, including cross-institutional adaptation and broader changes both within and exogenous to a society. The investigation of these variables can only be accomplished by longer-range historical analyses than those available in this book.

IMPLICATIONS FOR FAMILY RESEARCH AND THEORY

Featherman's (1985) definition of development in terms of duration and state dependence makes a great deal of intuitive sense. However, research in this area lags behind intuition, mainly because of the various logical problems that have plagued many of the conceptions of family stages.

It is doubtful that a truly accurate picture of family development will emerge unless we shift our focus from the individual as a unit of observation to the family group (stage) as a unit of analysis. Difficulties do arise when we consider the problem of who is to be the informant for each family—the mother, the father, or the child. As Chapter 8 points out, spouses' perceptions are seldom uniform. Elsewhere (White, 1984a), I have proposed that family members be treated as any other observers of a group. Thus, if any two family members are asked to report on events for a period of time, their reports should be checked for interobserver reliability, just as the reports of any other two observers of the same phenomenon are checked. In regard to the order and timing of major life events, there will be little discrepancy between these two reports (e.g., see Chapter 6); however, with less salient events or events salient to one individual but not to the others, recall may be quite different from family member to family member.

Although the present work has proposed a set of family stages, it remains for other theoreticians to develop a set of theoretical stages that fit the various *relationships* within the family, such as parent–child and sibling relationships. The fact that such relationships continue to develop outside the context of the family is not surprising. This, however, is a much more important insight as family-type relationships multiply with divorce and stepparenting. The fact that these relationships may not continue in the household in which the parent–child bond continues implies that they are not properly within the family group. Sometimes these relationships are between families (Ahrons & Rodgers, 1987). These relationships continue to develop over the life course of the dyad or triad. For example, the sibling relationship is by definition added some time after the beginning of the family unit and continues to develop long after the family group has ceased to exist. Because these relationships are kinship relations, one should not be led to the conclusion that they indicate the presence of a particular family. Some family relationships, such as sibling relationships, invariably outlive the family group in which they started. The challenge facing theorists is to specify the mutually exclusive and exhaustive stages for these family subgroup relationships. Only then will it be possible to see which stages of relationship development are dependent on particular family stages and their duration.

One implication of the present research is that it is not well advised to make claims about invariant family stages and monotonic family or relationship development. It is far better to discuss the entropy measure for a given family stage and to compare transition probabilities for leaving a given stage and moving to various next stages. Thus, a monotonic system of family stages may be characterized as a system in which each stage has low entropy and the transition probability for the next low entropy stage approaches 1. However, as I have previously mentioned, such a lockstep process of family development is probably only found in nursery rhymes, or perhaps in totalitarian societies. The research presented in this book clearly fails to support the conceptualization of an invariant and monotonic progression of family stages.

Another implication for researchers is that research on the topic of family change should specify what kind of change is meant and to which meaning of the family (institution or group) it pertains. Developmental change (within the institution, the family, or the individual) is change in which the stage and duration of the stage determine the probability for the subsequent stage. Evolutionary change (as natural selection) is mainly tied to the process of adaptation between institutions. The pressure for adaptation is revealed among individuals in cases where the individuals follow the norms of different institutions, but in doing so they experience an accumulation of too many events and expectations in too short a period of time. At the individual level this is recognized as stress; however, the etiology is at the institutional level and not at the individual level, as is often erroneously supposed by those attempting to help people adapt to unreasonable normative expectations. As the aggregate of individuals change their behavior to follow the norms of one institution and deviate from those in another, the norms of one institution are changed. This is a process of institutional adaptation (natural selection), since the institution must respond to such pressures or become extinct. Of course, most of the changes in family norms are of a less dramatic nature.

Social groups change mainly through their own developmental processes, which are in turn governed by social institutions. Social institutions change mainly through the process of adaptation to other institutions. No doubt some institutional change responds to pressures external to a particular social system, such as the worldwide pressure for more education and technology. Also, there is probably some change that is largely random or haphazard.

Family transitions are part of the developmental process of the family group. The family group is inextricably tied to the social changes within the social institution of the family, since the norms that regulate family stages are institutional norms. Since these institutional norms adapt to changes within other social institutions and to changes exogenous to the particular social system, family change cannot be fully understood without including these institutional and cross-institutional levels of analysis. The concept of family stages, as discussed in this chapter, links together the group structure and institutional norms to form meaningful categories for the analysis of family development. The fact that the individual actor plays little role in social change is not surprising. Indeed, the emphasis on the individual as the primary level of conceptual analysis in relation to family group phenomena has perhaps done more to retard a theory of family development than any other single form of influence. This work has attempted to reduce this effect.

ACKNOWLEDGMENTS

Much of this chapter owes a debt to discussions with Roy H. Rodgers. Furthermore, I would like to acknowledge helpful input from students in the Family Development Seminar, Department of Family Sciences, University of British Columbia: Marlene Atleo, Michelle Filion, Dolores Fischer, and Ilona Stigrad. The ideas expressed in this chapter are my sole responsibility.

NOTES

1. Note that the dynamic model of the theory is stochastic and not a deterministic cause-and-effect model.

2. Stages are generated as permutations on the set of three binary relations: affinal–consanguineal, male–female, and within–outside the domicile. For any specific society, there may be some theoretically possible stage with no empirical cases. Transition events can be society-specific.

3. See Stone (1988, p. 22, Chart 1.2) for an example of the relationship between family age and family diversity

CHAPTER 12

Epilogue

This epilogue takes a brief look back at how the basic questions regarding the theory have been addressed, and assesses the scientific and theoretical status of the theory of family development in comparison to some of the other theories about the family.

In Chapter 2, I have stated that this book is part of the continuing process of theory construction and refinement in the area of family development. It may now seem somewhat contradictory to make claims about the theoretical status of family development theory when I have been engaged in a process. However, in order to tie together the themes in this book, it is necessary to take a point-in-time snapshot of where the theory now stands and what has been accomplished. This assessment of the theory should not be interpreted as any form of closure for the theory or as any discouragement of continued theory construction and refinement.

BASIC QUESTIONS

At the outset of this book, I have noted that four areas cited by Mattessich and Hill (1987) did not receive adequate attention from earlier developmental theorists. At this point, it is fair to ask, "What progress has been made in relation to these four areas?"

1. *A single modal life cycle?* The first major criticism is that earlier scholars focused only on family stages in the modal life course pattern. A very important contributing factor to this exclusive focus on modal stages has been the lack of exhaustive and exclusive stages. Instead, most of the stage conceptions dealt with only the popular or modal stages and neglected others. This work has attempted to address this problem by proposing the structural–event approach to family stages discussed in the preceding chapter.

2. *Timing of critical life events.* The second criticism is that earlier versions of the theory ignored the timing and duration of critical life events. As pointed out at the beginning of this book, addressing this problem demands that the theorist clarify and define the relationship between "stage" and "event." This has been done in Chapter 3. In Chapter 4, a model is developed that incorporates the notion of *duration* in a stage as a significant component of the process of development. Chapters 7 and 8 have used empirical examples of how duration is used in the study of development. In a broader perspective, this criticism has been addressed by emphasizing the dynamic and processual parts of the theory. Previously, the dynamics of the theory were not well developed.

3. *The interaction effect of other careers.* The third major criticism is that the synchronization of the family career with careers in other sectors, such as work and education, was not addressed. In this work, by contrast, the coordination (or lack thereof) of norms between various institutions has been one of the principal topics. For example, a timing norm may suggest that one should marry in his or her early 20s, but this marital norm may conflict with work and education norms that stress staying in school for longer periods of time and getting a job before marriage. In addition, this work has suggested the importance of cross-institutional norms that coordinate timing and sequencing norms between institutions. Deviation from these institutional and cross-institutional norms is one of the ways in which institutional and societal change progresses.

4. *Lack of correlation with other measures.* The problem that the stages of the family proposed by earlier theorists have shown only very modest correlations with dependent variables is the last problem area cited by Mattessich and Hill (1987). In the perspective of this book, such low correlations should be expected when independent and dependent measures are from different levels of analysis, process is confused with point in time studies, and the very concept of "stages" is in need of revision. Once these areas of confusion are cleared up, there are undoubtedly some dependent variables affected by the attributes of particular family stages, and these can indeed be established by correlational research. However, this is using only the static aspect of the theory (roles and role relationships). The processual aspects of the theory of family development have only begun to receive attention (e.g., Menaghan, 1989). In this work, Chapters 7 and 8 have illustrated that transition probabilities are dependent upon both the family stage and the duration of time in that stage. Furthermore, the analysis of the norms of the family as an *institution* has for too long been sacrificed to discussions about individual-level roles. Chapters 9 and 10 suggest that the analysis of sequencing norms

both within an institution and between institutions may add to our understanding of how family development is woven into the fabric of a complex set of social institutions.

THEORETICAL STATUS

The claim that the theory of family development is indeed a scientific *theory* may seem bold to some and premature to others. Indeed, in Chapter 2, the process in this book has been identified as theory *construction*. I continue to believe that theories are always being refined and elaborated. Only at a point in time can we take a snapshot of the theory and ask whether it resembles a scientific theory. However, in the context of the history and maturation of these ideas, the claim for theoretical status seems simply overdue at this particular point in time. This appears all the more evident when we compare the theory of family development with other extant theories about the family.

Although scholars may quibble about the appropriate definition for a scientific theory, it would seem that the definition by Rudner (1966) is quite adequate: a set of systematically related propositions, containing some lawlike generalizations, which is empirically testable. This definition, adopted at the outset, has guided the present work on family development theory. There are three main components to this definition: A theory should be characterized by systematic relations, should contain some lawlike statements, and should be empirically testable. Each of these deserves separate consideration.

Systematic Relations

The theory of family development as it stands cannot be considered to be fully systematized. It does contain some systematic relations; for example, the definition of the process of development and the model appear to be relatively isomorphic. The definitional structure, especially for terms such as "position," "norm," "role," and "role relationship," is systematic. However, the concept of "family stages" has been problematic. Of all the concepts in the theory of family development, the stages concept *à la* Duvall is the most deeply embedded in the community of family scholars. This popular conception of stages fails to provide categories that are exclusive and exhaustive. The structural approach proposed in Chapter 11 resolves many of these problems and is consistent with the definitional structure.

Lawlike Generalizations

The theory as proposed in this work contains some lawlike generalizations. A "lawlike statement" is one in which two concepts are related in the same way as their corresponding measures are related, and the relation between these measures is invariant under certain specifiable conditions. For instance, the theory proposes that the present family stage and the duration of time in that stage determine the probabilities for stage transitions. The concepts in this proposition can be measured in terms of the aggregate frequencies for moving from one state to another, or in terms of the frequencies for an event at time 1, given another event at time 2. The boundary conditions for this relation are that the process is homogeneous in regard to the population and that no world crisis such as war or depression exists (all else being equal).

Empirically Testable

The last criterion for a scientific theory is that the set of statements must be empirically testable. Although the example above demonstrates that the theory is testable, there are other examples as well. Even the basic assumptions of the theory, such as the proposition that sequencing norms regulate family stage transitions, may be examined empirically. In order to test this proposition, sequencing norms must be measured as rules at time 1 when the family is in a particular stage. These rules regarding family sequencing can be measured both in terms of social expectations carried by individuals (as was previously accomplished by Neugarten et al., 1965) and in terms of aggregate-level behaviors (either the structural stage sequences or event sequences approximating these norms). The relation that would be expected between the individual normative expectations and the sequencing of family stages at the aggregate level would be that they are identical, except for variation created by sampling and measurement error. These sequencing norms would then be used to predict later family behavior.

This example brings up a potential criticism of the theory. It could appear to some that the theory is tautological,[1] and hence not empirically disconfirmable. Critics could argue that norms in this theory have two dimensions, expectations and behavior. At the aggregate level, the theory uses the modal behavior patterns (sequences) to infer the norms that are operating. These critics would then maintain that the theory falls into tautological reasoning when it attempts to explain these behavioral patterns as being caused by norms.

In order to address the concerns of such critics, we must have a better understanding of the nature of tautology and of when it is problematic for scientific theory. The common understanding is that a tautology exists when a statement is true by definition. However, since much of mathematical and logical inference could be considered to be tautological by this definition, we need to specify more clearly what "tautology" means. Rudner (1966) calls such systems of thought "analytical schemata." According to Rudner, such schemata all share the characteristic feature of "being able to be validated solely by recourse to the definitions of the system and logic, and not, as are empirical hypotheses, by recourse to any extralinguistic (empirical) investigations of evidence" (1966, p. 31). The major problem with logical systems is not that they are untrue, but that they do not represent scientific theories because they do not offer any propositions that might possibly be empirically disconfirmed. In order for a theory to be a *scientific* theory, it must have at least one such empirically disconfirmable proposition.

However, the theory of family development does offer many such propositions. One of the most obvious is the proposition that social norms change as a result of systematic behavioral deviance over time (Modell, 1980). Furthermore, the theory identifies norms as modal behavior at the aggregate level, with the recognition that this may be validated by the second dimension (expectations) also being present. When both are present, we have a valid picture of the timing (duration) and sequencing (stage) norms. These norms are then used to estimate the transition probabilities for the model of the developmental process. These transition probabilities are what help us make predictions. So, clearly, the theory enables predictions to be made from the norms at Time 1, then to estimate the parameters (probabilities) of the model, and finally to predict the probable behavioral paths at time 2. It is not tautological to say that the norms about timing and sequencing at time 1 predict the behavior of families at a later time. Indeed, this cannot be tautological, since the content of family norms at time 1 can vary independently of the normative content at time 2 and in no way are dictated by or derived from the analytical schemata of the theory.

According to this perspective, the theory of family development, though far from finished or complete, does approximate what we expect in a scientific theory. The next question is this: "How does the theory of family development compare with other theories about families?"

OTHER THEORIES ABOUT FAMILIES

When scholars talk about either family change or family continuity, they must consider comparisons between family structures over time. This fact should alert theorists to the importance of the time dimension in any theory about the family. However, the theory of family development is the only one that conscientiously deals with the time dimension. Other family theories, such as symbolic interaction or exchange theory, do not deal well with the concepts of time and process. In fact, there is no clear statement specifying processes of change in families in most of the other extant theories. A few theories, such as conflict theory, may make some claim that they discuss processes (e.g., dialectical processes), but these are seldom specified in any detail or with any precision.

Other theories also do not connect well with the broader institutional fabric of the social system. Most of the other theories about the family fail to fill in the gap between the behavior of the group and the institutions of the social system. The fact that the theory of family development deals with the relationships between and among individual, relationship, group, institutional, and cross-institutional levels reveals its breadth and potential connectedness to broader theories of social structure and change.

Other theories fail to consider that propositions must be appropriate for the level of analysis, at least in part because they take the individual as ultimately the only "real" level of analysis. This is what Featherman (1985) labels the "personological bias" in developmental research. Certainly, the theory of family development is not exempt from this criticism. However, since the work by Rodgers (1973), at least some formulations of the theory have moved away from this exclusive focus on the individual.

Finally, the theory of family development is more precise than other theories about the family. This precision comes in large part from the formalization of the developmental process in the model. No other extant theories about the family have attempted formalization or suggested the relationship between theory and a specific model.[2] Since family development theory is more formally developed, it is inherently more easily disconfirmed, since the claim that data fit a particular model is more stringent than in theories where data are generalized by some model.

The future for the theory of family development depends on a continuation of its popular appeal, coupled with continuing systematic structuring. The theory of family development will continue to have a following because of the intuitive appeal of the stages concept. The process part of the theory needs to receive greater amounts of attention from those scholars interested in social change as a many-leveled process. There should also be renewed emphasis on the collection of data units of analysis other than the individual. Despite the many aspects of the theory in need of attention, it stands as one of the best-developed and most precise theories about family structure and change. Its status in this regard can only improve as scholars join the process of refining this multileveled theory about the ways in which families traverse their life course.

SUMMING UP

This book has emphasized the dynamic aspects of the theory of family development. Previous scholars have addressed the role structure and role relationships within particular modal stages of family development (e.g., Rodgers, 1973; Aldous, 1978). The discussion presented here does not discount previous microstructural approaches, but rather complements them in several ways. For example, the present work supplies a clearer notion of some concepts, such as stages and positions in the family.

The dynamic process of family development has been characterized by some as a teleological process. For example, Mattessich and Hill (1987) suggest that it is a process moving toward greater structural differentiation. This type of claim may have originated from borrowing the idea of development often used in child psychology. The problem is that this teleological notion of development fails to be very convincing in either a life span perspective on individuals or a life course perpective on families. Indeed, it only makes sense if we truncate the process of development by stipulating that it ends with the ending of childhood. However, most adults feel that they, too, continue to develop.

The approach taken in this book is that family development is a stochastic or probabilistic process. It is not a lockstep, deterministic process aimed at some teleological goal. However, explanation is possible without teleology. The process of family development is defined as one in which the probability of a transition to another stage depends on the stage currently occupied and the duration of time spent in that stage. The explanation of why this is so is that each social system contains norms about the sequencing and timing of family stages. These family processual norms suggest how stages are sequenced, as well as how much time is spent in a stage before a transition is appropriate. For example, the sequencing norms suggest that the stage of "newly married couple" be followed by the event of the birth of the first child or the "early family" stage. Timing norms suggest that a newly married couple wait a year or two before having children, but not 10 or 20 years. In other words, the sequencing norms establish the stage transition dependencies, and the timing norms establish the duration dependencies.

Although families in North America predominantly follow the modal or normatively established path, there is some variation. Some of this is random variation, and some is systematic nonconformity to the family sequencing and timing norms. This systematic nonconformity or deviance is often explainable by the fact that the sequencing and timing norms of the institution of the family are not coordinated with the processual norms of other social institutions. In such cases, families and individuals systematically deviate from one set of norms in order to conform to another set.

The family processual norms change over time as a result of this process of cross-institutional adaptation. Therefore, over time we can expect changes in the normative path of family development within a social system. As a further consequence of this process of adaptation, we can expect that some previously non-normative stages of family development may evolve to become modal and expected, and that some older stages may devolve and become less traveled and non-normative. Therefore, the modal path identified at one point in history is unlikely to be identical to one at a much later point.

It is undoubtedly true that all cultures have their own family norms; it is simultaneously true that some family norms, such as nuclear-family incest taboos, are cross-culturally uniform. World system pressures, such as information exchange and economic exchange, suggest that the similarity in family processual norms may be increasing (Kumagai, 1984). The entropy measure suggested in Chapter 11 offers a way of computing changes in family stage behavior that may be used to compare different time points within a culture or two distinct cultures. It is important to recognize, however, that historical and cross-cultural comparisons depend on a relatively abstract and universally applicable set of family stages.

This work opens many questions and avenues for thought and research. For instance, the exact parameters for the process of deviance and conformity are not yet established. When family norms do not coordinate with work norms, does deviance always result in the family arena and conformity usually result in the work world? If economic values and goals are more salient than family values, then indeed this might be the case. However, this argument that the institution of the family is largely the effect rather than the cause of such changes does not seem supported in North America, where employers are gradually instituting on-site day care facilities and family leave time as routine parts of the work environment. Researchers and theorists might also explore the gender differences in cross-institutional norms. It is probably true that males and females follow the same family processual norms.

However, these family timing and sequencing norms developed in a previous period, when work and education norms were seen as less salient for women. Undoubtedly, changes in the cross-institutional normative fabric require adaptations in the timing and sequencing of the family, work, and education careers.

Finally, many questions abound about the rate of change in the institution of the family, compared to the rate of change in other social institutions. For instance, the question "Will the family survive?" is predicated on the notion that the institution of the family changes more than do other social institutions. For family scholars, this question can be partially addressed by examining the rate and direction of systematic deviance in our social institutions. If indeed there is less conformity to family processual and static norms than to work or educational norms, then clearly the family is less salient as an institution in that social system.

The theory of family development cannot answer all of the questions about family change. Some changes are random; other changes are the result of cross-institutional adaptation. But some changes are developmental in nature. These developmental changes, and the conditions that drive them, are what the theory of family development attempts to explain.

NOTES

1. I wish to thank David Klein for raising this as a possible criticism of the theory.

2. Exchange and equity theories may offer some formal models for balancing resources, exchanges, rewards, and so on, but such models are usually restricted to dyads and are not applicable to family groups.

References

Ahrons, C., & Rodgers, R. H. (1987). *Divorced families.* New York: Norton.

Aldous, J. (1978). *Family careers.* New York: Wiley.

Allison, P. D. (1984). *Event history analysis: Regression for longitudinal event data* (Sage University Paper Series on Quantitative Applications in the Social Sciences, No. 07-046). Beverly Hills, CA: Sage.

Anderson, S. A., Russell, C. S., & Schumm, W. R. (1983). Perceived marital quality and family life-cycle categories: A further analysis. *Journal of Marriage and the Family, 45,* 127–139.

Baltes, P. B. (1968). Longitudinal and cross-sectional sequences in the study of age and generation effects. *Human Development, 11,* 145–171.

Baltes, P. B., & Schaie, K. W. (Eds.). (1973). *Life-span developmental psychology: Personality and socialization.* New York: Academic Press.

Bates, F. L. (1956). Position, role and status: A reformulation of concepts. *Social Forces, 34,* 313–321.

Bengtson, V. L. (1975). Generation and family effects in value socialization. *American Sociological Review, 40,* 358–371.

Bierstedt, R. (1970). *The social order.* New York: McGraw-Hill.

Black, M. (1962). *Models and metaphors.* Ithaca, NY: Cornell University Press.

Borne, H., Jache, A., & Sederberg, N., with Klein, D. M. (1979). *Family chronogram analysis: Toward the development of new methodological tools for assessing the life cycles of families.* Paper presented at the Theory Construction and Methodology Workshop, National Council on Family Relations, Boston.

Bronfenbrenner, U. (1979). *The ecology of human development.* Cambridge, MA: Harvard University Press.

Brooks, D. R., & Wiley, E. O. (1986). *Evolution as entropy: Toward a unified theory of biology.* Chicago: University of Chicago Press.

Burch, T. K. (1985, August) *Family History Survey* (Statistics Canada, Catalogue No. 99-955). Ottawa: Statistics Canada.

Burch, T. K., & Madan, A. K. (1986). *Union formation and dissolution* (Statistics Canada, Catalogue No. 99-963). Ottawa: Statistics Canada.

Burr, W. R. (1970). *Theory construction and the sociology of the family.* New York: Wiley.

Caplow, T. (1968). *Two against one: Coalitions in triads*. Englewood Cliffs, NJ: Prentice-Hall.

Cherlin, A., & Horvich, S. (1980). Retrospective reports of family structure: A methodological assessment. *Sociological Methods of Research, 8,* 454–469.

Coleman, J. S. (1964). *Introduction to mathematical sociology*. New York: Free Press.

Coleman, J. S. (1981). *Longitudinal data analysis*. New York: Basic Books.

Cox, D. R. (1972). Regression models and life tables. *Journal of the Royal Statistical Society, Series B, 34,* 187–202.

Cox, D. R. (1975). Partial likelihood. *Biometrika, 62,* 269–276.

Cronbach, L. J. (1958). Proposals leading to analytic treatment of social perception scores. In R. Taguiri & L. Petrullo (Eds.), *Person perception and interpersonal behavior* (pp. 353–378). Stanford, CA: Stanford University Press.

Datan, N. (1983). Normative or not?: Confessions of a fallen epistemologist. In E. J. Callahan & K. A. McKluskey (Eds.), *Life-span developmental psychology: Non-normative life events* (pp. 35–43). New York: Academic Press.

Duvall, E. (1971). *Family development* (4th ed.). Philadelphia: J. B. Lippincott.

Duvall, E., & Hill, R. (1948). *Report of the Committee on the Dynamics of Family Interaction*. Paper presented at the National Conference on Family Life, Washington, DC.

Dymond, R. (1954). Interpersonal perception and marital happiness. *Canadian Journal of Psychology, 8,* 164–171.

Eichler, M. (1988). *Families in Canada today* (2nd ed.). Toronto: Gage.

Elder, G. H., Jr. (1974). *Children of the Great Depression*. Chicago: University of Chicago Press.

Elder, G. H., Jr. (1978). Approaches to social change and the family. *American Journal of Sociology, 84* (Suppl.), S1–S38.

Elder, G. H., Jr. (Ed.). (1985). *Life course dynamics: Trajectories and transitions, 1968–1980*. Ithaca, NY: Cornell University Press.

Elder, G. H., Jr. (1987). Families and lives: Some developments in life-course studies. *Journal of Family History, 12,* 179–199.

Farber, B. (1961). The family as a set of mutually contingent careers. In N. Foote (Ed.), *Consumer behavior: Models of household decision making* (pp. 276–297). New York: New York University Press.

Featherman, D. L. (1980). Retrospective longitudinal research: Methodological considerations. *Journal of Economics and Business, 32,* 152–169.

Featherman, D. L. (1985). Individual development and aging as a population process. In J. Nesselroade & A. von Eye (Eds.), *Individual development and social change: Exploratory analysis* (pp. 213–241). New York: Academic Press.

Feldman, H., & Feldman, M. (1975). The family life cycle: Some suggestions for recycling. *Journal of Marriage and the Family, 37,* 277–284.

Ferber, M. A., & Birnbaum, B. G. (1979). Retrospective earnings data: Some solutions for old problems. *Public Opinion Quarterly, 43,* 112–118.

Fincham, F. D., & Bradbury, T. N. (1987). The assessment of marital quality: A reevaluation. *Journal of Marriage and the Family, 49,* 797–810.

Finney, H. C. (1981). Improving the reliability of retrospective survey measures: Results of a longitudinal field survey. *Evaluation Quarterly, 5,* 207–229.

Flament, C. (1963). *Applications of graph theory to group structure.* Englewood Cliffs, NJ: Prentice-Hall.

Flavell, J. H. (1963). *The developmental psychology of Jean Piaget.* Princeton, NJ: Van Nostrand.

Gibbs, J. P. (1965). Norms: The problem of definition and classification. *American Journal of Sociology, 70,* 586–594.

Glenn, N. D. (1977). *Cohort analysis* (Sage University Paper Series on Quantitative Applications in the Social Sciences, No. 07-005). Beverly Hills, CA: Sage.

Glenn, N. D., & Kramer, K. B. (1987). The marriages and divorces of the children of divorce. *Journal of Marriage and the Family, 49,* 822–826.

Glick, P. C. (1947). The family cycle. *American Sociological Review, 12,* 164–174.

Glick, P. C. (1977). Updating the life cycle of the family. *Journal of Marriage and the Family, 39,* 5–13.

Goodman, L. (1972). A modified multiple regression approach to the analysis of dichotomous variables. *American Sociological Review, 37,* 28–46.

Gottman, J. M. (1979). *Marital interaction: Experimental investigations.* New York: Academic Press.

Gottman, J. M., & Porterfield, A. L. (1981). Communicative competence in the nonverbal behavior of married couples. *Journal of Marriage and the Family, 42,* 817–824.

Gross, N., Mason, W. S., & McEachern, A. W. (1958). *Explorations in role analysis.* New York: Wiley.

Gutek, B. A. (1978). On the accuracy of retrospective attitudinal data. *Public Opinion Quarterly, 42,* 390–401.

Gwartney-Gibbs, P. A. (1986). The institutionalization of premarital cohabitation: Estimates from marriage license applications, 1970 and 1980. *Journal of Marriage and the Family, 48,* 423–434.

Hannan, M. T., & Freeman, J. (1977). The population ecology of organizations. *American Journal of Sociology, 82,* 929–964.

Hannan, M. T., & Freeman, J. (1984). Structural inertia and organizational change. *American Sociological Review, 49,* 149–64.

Hareven, T. K. (1978). Cycles, courses and cohorts: Reflections on theoretical and methodological approaches to the historical study of family development. *Journal of Social History, 12,* 97–109.

Havighurst, R. J. (1948). *Developmental tasks and education.* New York: David McKay.

Hawley, A. (1950). *Human ecology: A theory of community structure.* New York: Ronald Press.

Henry, J. (1964). *Jungle people.* New York: Vintage Books.

Hill, R. (1986). Life cycle stages for types of single parent families. *Family Relations, 35,* 19–29.

Hill, R., & Hansen, D. A. (1960). The identification of conceptual frameworks utilized in family study. *Marriage and Family Living, 22,* 299–311.

Hill, R., & Mattessich, P. (1979). Family development theory and life span development. In P. B. Baltes & O. Brim (Eds.), *Life span development and behavior* (Vol. 2, pp. 161–204). New York: Academic Press.

Hill, R., & Mederer, H. (1983). Critical transitions over the life span: Theory and research. In H. McCubbin, M. Sussman, & J. Patterson (Eds.), *Social stress and the family: Advances in family stress theory and research* (pp. 271–321). New York: Haworth Press.

Hill, R., & Rodgers, R. H. (1964). The developmental approach. In H. T. Christensen (Ed.), *Handbook of marriage and the family* (pp. 171–211). Chicago: Rand McNally.

Hogan, D. P. (1978). The variable order of events in the life course. *American Sociological Review, 43,* 573–586.

Hogan, D. P. (1981). *Transitions and social change: The early lives of American men.* New York: Academic Press.

Hogan, D. P., & Astone, N. M. (1986). The transition to adulthood. *Annual Review of Sociology, 12,* 109–130.

Homans, G. C. (1967). *The nature of social science.* New York: Harcourt, Brace & World.

Hull, C. H., & Nie, N. H. (Eds.) (1979). *SPSS Update: New procedures and facilities for releases 7 and 8.* New York: McGraw Hill.

Kelley, H. H., Berscheid, E., Christensen, A., Harvey, J. H., Huston, T. L., Levinger, G., McClintock, E., Peplau, L. A., & Pederson, D. R. (Eds.). (1983). *Close relationships.* New York: W. H. Freeman.

Kemeny, J. G., Mirkil, H., Snell, J. L., & Thompson, G. L. (1958). *Finite mathematical structures.* Englewood Cliffs, NJ: Prentice-Hall.

Kerlinger, F. N. (1973). *Foundations of behavioral research* (2nd ed.). New York: Holt, Rinehart & Winston.

Kirkpatrick, C., & Hobart, C. (1954). Disagreement, disagreement estimate, and non-empathic imputations for intimacy groups varying from favorite date to married. *American Sociological Review, 19,* 10–19.

Klein, D. M., & Aldous, J. (1979). Three blind mice: Criticisms of the "family life cycle" concept. *Journal of Marriage and the Family, 41,* 689–691.

Kuhn, T. S. (1962). *The structure of scientific revolutions.* Chicago: University of Chicago Press.

Kumagai, F. (1984). The life cycle of the Japanese family. *Journal of Marriage and the Family, 46,* 191–204.

Laing, R. D., Phillipson, H., & Lee, A. (1966). *Interpersonal perception.* New York: Springer.

Larson, L. E. (1974). System and subsystem perception of family roles. *Journal of Marriage and the Family, 36,* 123–138.

Lee, E., & Desu, M. (1972). A computer program for comparing K samples with right-censored data. *Computer Programs in Biomedicine, 2,* 315–321.

Leik, R. K., & Meeker, B. F. (1975). *Mathematical sociology.* Englewood Cliffs, NJ: Prentice-Hall.

Lévi-Strauss, C. (1949). *The elementary structures of kinship.* Boston: Beacon Press.

Lewis, R. A., & Spanier, G. B. (1979). Theorizing about the quality and stability of marriage. In W. R. Burr, R. Hill, F. I. Nye, & I. L. Reiss, (Eds.), *Contemporary theories about the family* (Vol. 1, pp. 268–294). New York: Free Press.

Magrabi, F. M., & Marshall, W. H. (1965). Family developmental tasks: A research model. *Journal of Marriage and the Family, 27,* 454–461.

Marini, M. M. (1984). Age and sequencing norms in the transition to adulthood. *Social Forces, 63,* 229–244.

Mattessich, P., & Hill, R. (1987). Life cycle and family development. In M. B. Sussman & S. Steinmetz (Eds.), *Handbook of marriage and the family* (pp. 437–469). New York: Plenum.

McLain, R., & Weigert, A. (1979). Toward a phenomenological sociology of family: A programmatic essay. In W. R. Burr, (Eds.), *Contemporary theories about the family* (Vol. 2, pp. 160–205). New York: Free Press.

Menaghan, E. (1983). Marital stress and family transitions: A panel analysis. *Journal of Marriage and the Family, 45,* 371–386.

Menaghan, E. (1989). Role changes and psychological well being: Variations in effects by gender and role repertoire. *Social Forces, 67,* 693–714.

Merton, R. K. (1949). *Social theory and social structure.* Glencoe, IL: Free Press.

Miller, S. A. (1987). *Developmental research methods.* Englewood Cliffs, NJ: Prentice-Hall.

Modell, J. (1980). Normative aspects of marriage timing since World War II. *Journal of Family History, 5,* 210–234.

Morgan, S. P., & Rindfuss, R. R. (1985). Marital disruption: Structural and temporal dimensions. *American Journal of Sociology, 90,* 1055–1077.

Murdock, G. P. (1949). *Social structure.* New York: Macmillan.

Neugarten, B. L., Moore, J. W., & Lowe, J. C. (1965). Age norms, age constraints, and adult socialization. *American Journal of Sociology, 70,* 710–717.

Niemi, R. G. (1974). *How family members perceive each other: Political and social attitudes in two generations.* New Haven, CT: Yale University Press.

Nock, S. (1979). The family life cycle: Empirical or conceptual tool? *Journal of Marriage and the Family, 41,* 15–26.

Noller, P. (1984). *Nonverbal communication and marital interaction.* New York: Pergamon Press.

Norton, R. (1983). Measuring marital quality: A critical look at the dependent variable. *Journal of Marriage and the Family, 45,* 141–151.

Parsons, T., & Bales, R. F. (1955). *Family, socialization and interaction processes.* New York: Free Press.

Pearlin, L. I. (1980). The life cycle and life strains. In H. Blalock, Jr. (Ed.), *Sociological theory and research: A critical appraisal* (pp. 349–360). NY: Free Press.

Pearlin, L. I., & Schooler, C. (1978). The structure of coping. *Journal of Health and Social Behavior, 19,* 2–21.

Popper, K. R. (1959). *The logic of scientific discovery.* New York: Basic Books.

Prigogene, I., & Stengers, I. (1984). *Order out of chaos.* New York: Bantam Books.

Reiss, I. L. (1965). The universality of the family: A conceptual analysis. *Journal of Marriage and the Family, 27,* 443–453.

Reiss, I. L., & Lee, G. R. (1988). *Family systems in America* (4th ed.). New York: Holt, Rinehart & Winston.

Rodgers, R. H. (1973). *Family interaction and transaction: The developmental approach.* Engelwood Cliffs, NJ: Prentice-Hall.

Rodgers, R. H., & Witney, G. (1981). The family cycle in twentieth century Canada. *Journal of Marriage and the Family, 43,* 727–740.

Rollins, B., & Feldman, H. (1970). Marital satisfaction over the family life cycle. *Journal of Marriage and the Family, 32,* 20–27.

Rudner, R. S. (1966). *Philosophy of social science.* Englewood Cliffs, NJ: Prentice-Hall.

Ryder, N. B. (1965). The cohort as a concept in the study of social change. *American Sociological Review, 30,* 843–861.

Schram, R. W. (1979). Marital satisfaction over the life cycle: A critique and a proposal. *Journal of Marriage and the Family, 41,* 7–14.

Schusky, E. L. (1965). *Manual for kinship analysis.* New York: Holt, Rinehart & Winston.

Spanier, G. B. (1976). Measuring dyadic adjustment: New scales for assessing the quality of marriage and similar dyads. *Journal of Marriage and the Family, 38,* 15–28.

Spanier, G. B., Sauer, W., & Larzelere, R. (1979). An empirical evaluation of the family life cycle. *Journal of Marriage and the Family, 41,* 27–38.

Statistics Canada. (1977). *Methodology of the Canadian Labour Force Survey,* 1976 (Statistics Canada, Catalogue No. 71-526). Ottawa: Author.

Stone, L. O. (1988). *Family and friendship ties among Canada's elderly* (Statistics Canada, Catalogue No. 89–508). Ottawa: Statistics Canada.

Teachman, J. D. (1982). Methodological issues in the analysis of family formation and dissolution. *Journal of Marriage and the Family, 44,* 1037–1053.

Teachman, J. D., & Polonko, K. A. (1984). Timing of the transition to parenthood: A multidimensional birth-interval approach. *Journal of Marriage and the Family, 47,* 867–880.

Tuma, N. B., & Hannan, M. T. (1984). *Social dynamics.* New York: Academic Press.

Waller, W., & Hill, R. (1951). *The family: A dynamic interpretation* (rev. ed.). New York: Dryden Press.

White, H. C. (1963). *An anatomy of kinship.* Englewood Cliffs, NJ: Prentice-Hall.

White, J. M. (1982). Dyadic systems analysis. *Behavioral Science, 27,* 104–117.

White, J. M. (1984a). Not the sum of its parts. *Journal of Family Issues, 5,* 515–518.

White, J. M. (1984b). A cohort analysis of the family career. *Journal of Comparative Family Studies, 15,* 29–41.

White, J. M. (1985). Perceived similarity and understanding in married couples. *Journal of Social and Personal Relationships, 2,* 45–57.

White, J. M. (1987a). Researching developmental careers: The Career Conformity Scale. *Journal of Family Issues, 8,* 306–318.

White, J. M. (1987b). Marital perceived agreement and actual agreement over the family life cycle. *Journal of Comparative Family Studies, 18,* 47–59.

White, J. M. (1988). Marriage: A developing process. In K. Ishwaran (Ed.), *The modern family: A cross-cultural introduction* (pp. 197–211). Toronto: Wall & Thompson.

White, J. M., & Reid, N. (1984). *Modelling the family career: Theoretical and methodological issues in the application of stochastic models to developmental theory of the family.* Paper presented at the meeting of the National Council on Family Relations, San Francisco.

Wilson, R. S. (1975). Analysis of developmental data: Comparison among alternative methods. *Developmental Psychology, 11,* 676–680.

Yarrow, M. R., Campbell, J. D., & Burton, R. V. (1970). Recollections of childhood: A study of the retrospective method. *Monographs of the Society for Research in Child Development, 35* (5, Serial No. 138).

Index